Fit for Duty

SECOND EDITION

Robert Hoffman
Thomas R. Collingwood

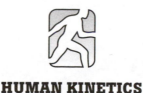

HUMAN KINETICS

Library of Congress Cataloging-in-Publication Data

Hoffman, Robert.
  Fit for duty / Robert Hoffman, Thomas R. Collingwood.--2nd ed.
      p. cm.
  Includes bibliographical references and index.
  ISBN 0-7360-5543-6 (soft cover : alk. paper)
  1. Police--Health and hygiene. 2. Physical fitness. I. Collingwood, Thomas R.
II. Title.
  HV7936.H4H627 2005
  613'.02'43632--dc22

                                                    2005013720

ISBN: 0-7360-5543-6

Acquisitions Editor: Michael S. Bahrke, PhD; **Developmental Editor:** Amanda S. Ewing; **Assistant Editor:** Bethany J. Bentley; **Copyeditor:** Barbara Field; **Proofreader:** Coree Clark; **Indexer:** Betty Frizzéll; **Permission Manager:** Dalene Reeder; **Graphic Designer:** Robert Reuther; **Graphic Artist:** Tara Welsch; **Photo Manager:** Dan Wendt; **Cover Designer:** Keith Blomberg; **Photographer (cover):** Dan Wendt; **Photographer (interior):** Dan Wendt, unless otherwise noted; **Art Manager:** Kareema McLendon; **Illustrator:** Argosy; **Printer:** Versa Press

We thank the Champaign Police Department in Champaign, Illinois, for assistance in providing the location for the photo shoot for this book.

Human Kinetics books are available at special discounts for bulk purchase. Special editions or book excerpts can also be created to specification. For details, contact the Special Sales Manager at Human Kinetics.

Printed in the United States of America   10   9   8   7   6   5   4   3   2   1

Human Kinetics
Web site: www.HumanKinetics.com

United States: Human Kinetics
P.O. Box 5076
Champaign, IL 61825-5076
800-747-4457
e-mail: humank@hkusa.com

Canada: Human Kinetics
475 Devonshire Road Unit 100
Windsor, ON N8Y 2L5
800-465-7301 (in Canada only)
e-mail: orders@hkcanada.com

Europe: Human Kinetics
107 Bradford Road
Stanningley
Leeds LS28 6AT, United Kingdom
+44 (0) 113 255 5665
e-mail: hk@hkeurope.com

Australia: Human Kinetics
57A Price Avenue
Lower Mitcham, South Australia 5062
08 8277 1555
e-mail: liaw@hkaustralia.com

New Zealand: Human Kinetics
Division of Sports Distributors NZ Ltd.
P.O. Box 300 226 Albany
North Shore City
Auckland
0064 9 448 1207
e-mail: info@humankinetics.co.nz

CONTENTS

PREFACE

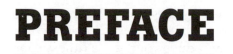

On February 6, 2005, players on the New England Patriots and Philadelphia Eagles football teams awoke knowing it was going to be a critical day—the day they had trained for their entire professional careers. They had watched film of their opponent, developed a game plan, and practiced against the scout team. They knew the game was going to kick off at 6:27 p.m. and last for four quarters of 15 minutes each. During the game, there were time-outs, a halftime break, substitutions, and specialists for certain situations. No player was in for more than half of the game. After the game, both the winners and the losers returned to their loved ones, and half of them celebrated a victory in arguably the biggest sporting event in America. Millions of people were glued to their televisions for the game, watched the postgame antics in the winning locker room, and listened to the losers express their disappointment.

On September 11, 2001, officers in the New York and New Jersey Port Authority and the New York City Police Departments awoke with absolutely *no* idea that it was *the* most critical day of their lives—the day they had trained for their entire careers. They had no film, no plan, no scout team. They didn't know what time the event was going to occur or how long it would last. There were no time-outs, no halftime break, no substitutions. Many of them did not return to their loved ones from the biggest terrorist attack the United States had ever experienced. Millions of Americans were glued to their televisions, and the images are forever burned in our memories. Officers assisting shocked victims to safety, carrying injured civilians and other officers, and finally running for their own lives as the towers sank into the New York pavement.

How prepared were those officers? How prepared are you if today is your Super Bowl? Will your level of fitness enable you to perform those tasks, or will you, your partner, and the public be in jeopardy because of your lack of fitness?

Since Human Kinetics published the first edition of *Fit for Duty* almost 10 years ago, the authors have continued to work with law enforcement agencies and individual officers across the country on fitness programs and issues. Sadly, despite the wake-up call of September 11, many are still unprepared for those infrequent but perhaps critical events. Their reasoning goes something like this: "I've been doing this job for a long time, and I haven't once been called on to do any of those things. Besides, my experience helps make up for my lack of fitness."

In most agencies, the only time officers have to demonstrate some level of fitness is when they are not yet even law enforcement officers. That is, to get into and graduate from an academy, candidates usually have to pass some sort of fitness test. Once they become officers, they are no longer held accountable for their physical fitness. Thus, if you are interested in improving your fitness, you will most likely be doing it on your own. So how can this book help you?

We've learned a lot more about law enforcement fitness issues in the past 10 years and have made some significant changes to this book. In addition to updated statistics and anecdotes, we have expanded the chapters that teach you how to train for each component of fitness. In particular, we've included additional training modalities for anaerobic fitness, as we've learned more about the importance of that fitness component for law enforcement officers. For those of you who have been sedentary for a while, chapter 2, "How Do You Get Started?," may reduce your anxiety about beginning a fitness program. The chapters on diet and nutrition and goal setting have likewise been changed to make them more user-friendly, especially for the beginner.

Helping officers attain adequate levels of fitness to perform their essential job functions at a minimum level of safety and effectiveness is still the primary purpose of this book. But we know that it is not just exercise that gets officers fit enough to perform. What they eat, how they manage their weight and their stress, and whether or not they use tobacco and abuse substances such as alcohol and drugs affect their fitness for duty. Together with exercise, these lifestyle choices have a bearing on longevity and quality of life—two areas in which law enforcement officers tend to fall below the national norms. So this edition of the book again promotes a total fitness approach.

Although the principles of fitness are the same for everyone (regardless of profession), this book looks at each element of a fitness program from a law enforcement viewpoint. It is based on 40 years of law enforcement fitness experience, as well as feedback from numerous law enforcement officers from around the country. The principles have been put into practice repeatedly in the field and found to produce the desired results. The book focuses on physical fitness and will help you develop an individual exercise plan to either improve or maintain your current level of physical fitness. Since the other components of total fitness interrelate with physical fitness and with each other, you will learn the basics of each component and where to go if you need additional help.

This doesn't mean that what you learn about fitness is specific only to law enforcement officers. The lessons you learn here can be shared with your family and friends. You'll be doing them a favor while you help yourself.

To get the most out of this book, you must interact with it. It contains numerous exercises and some forms to complete. Some of you may be doing these exercises under the direction of a fitness coordinator; others will be participating on your own. The book is designed to help you succeed either way.

The book will also help you design your own individualized exercise program. You'll learn how to assess your current fitness level so you'll know where to begin, then how to set your goals for maintenance or improvement. You can use this book to develop a program that will challenge you whether you are already fit or just a beginner.

Most important, this book goes beyond merely telling you what to do; it tells you how and why. By reading this book, you will increase your knowledge of fitness as well as improve your fitness and health.

ORGANIZATION OF THE TEXT

Part I of the book sets the stage for the rest of the book. Chapter 1 discusses why fitness is important to law enforcement officers. We've provided updated information on the physical demands of law enforcement work based on studies we have conducted with more than 100 agencies during the past 10 years. We believe a key addition to this book is chapter 2, "How Do You Get Started?" As mentioned earlier, this chapter will allay the fears of previously sedentary officers by emphasizing the importance of moderation and progression when making the decision to improve your fitness. It also discusses options for being more active while performing what is largely a sedentary job. Chapter 3 helps you to assess your own fitness and compare your performance to other officers using updated normative fitness data.

Part II is an explanation of physical fitness, including a description of its components: how to design a program and evaluate progress. The chapters cover the principles of exercise, cardiovascular endurance conditioning, muscular strength and endurance conditioning, flexibility, and anaerobic fitness. We've expanded the chapter on resistance training and included sample programs for improving push-ups and the vertical jump. You may be pleasantly surprised to learn that attaining and maintaining requisite levels of fitness can be accomplished with as few as three hours of training per week.

Part III discusses the lifestyle components of fitness. This part teaches you how certain lifestyle choices affect your health as well as your job performance and where to go for additional help, if needed. It includes chapters on nutrition, weight management, stress management, smoking cessation, and substance abuse prevention. We'll help you sort through the myths and facts concerning the numerous fad diets currently in vogue, explain why exercise is the best stress-management tool, and steer you in the right direction if you are having trouble with your other lifestyle habits.

The other key to improving health and performance is behavioral change, which is covered in part IV. You'll determine where you stand on the scale of readiness for change. The process of changing behavior is not hard to understand but can be difficult to implement. This book will teach you how to make the necessary changes. It will show you how to assess your current fitness level, educate you about training plans, and teach you how to set goals.

By reading this far, you have indicated a desire to improve your fitness. The cost to you is a little time. The payoff is substantial. In addition to the benefits noted above, you will look better, feel better about yourself, reduce the stress in your life, and live a longer, better life. You may not have faced any of the situations requiring fitness thus far in your career, but there is no guarantee you won't have to today or tomorrow. Will you be ready? To improve your chances, turn to chapter 1 and get started! In the long run, you'll be glad you did.

ACKNOWLEDGMENTS

We are indebted to many people for helping us publish this book. Obviously, it couldn't have been done without the loyal efforts of the editorial and production staffs at Human Kinetics. We'd also like to thank the thousands of law enforcement officers across the United States who have inspired us with their devotion to protecting and serving their communities, their states, and our country. We are also grateful to Jay Smith, president of FitForce, for his review and valuable feedback. Last, but certainly not least, our continued gratitude to Barbara and Gretchen, our comptrollers, travel agents, and sounding boards, for their support and love.

Assessing Your Fitness

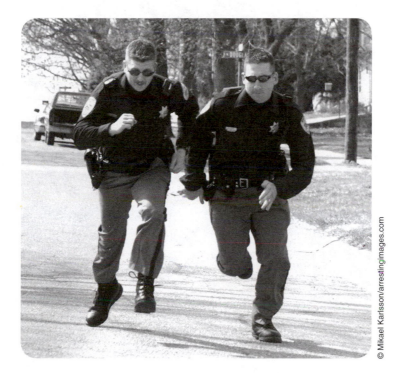

© Mikael Karlsson/arrestingimages.com

ealth and physical fitness are timely and popular topics. Every day we hear some news item reporting the results of recent health- or fitness-related research, and the news is rarely good: "Rising levels of obesity" or "More children are physically inactive" or "Sedentary living and poor nutrition are overtaking smoking as the biggest killers in America." Although occasionally the new information conflicts with earlier reports, the research is clear on one point: Lifestyle choices that people make every day have a significant bearing on their performance and health.

In the first edition of this book, we stated that the public is much more aware of and concerned with health and fitness than ever before. Now we're not so sure. This concern with health and fitness has been equally ambivalent within law enforcement agencies. Visionary administrators, as well as some individual officers, have come to realize that an officer who is fit will perform better, be healthier, and cost the agency less money in sick time, disability, and liability. Others have been dragging their feet, apparently not convinced that the job requires some degree of physical fitness.

Although agencies can't require officers to be healthy because of the Americans With Disabilities Act, they can require that they be able to perform critical physical tasks at a minimum level of safety and effectiveness. The good news is that you don't have to choose between the two. If you make lifestyle choices to improve your performance, you will realize the health benefits as well.

Fitness has become a concern for agencies in that officer physical readiness is now viewed as an important personnel issue. With the recognition since September 11 that a law enforcement officer is often the critical first responder, your fitness is not just your concern but your agency's and the public's as well. The fact that you are reading this book probably means that either you have come to this realization yourself or your agency has provided you an opportunity to improve your fitness by launching a fitness program. In either case, the first part of this book is important to your overall understanding of the issue.

The purpose of part I is to give you general information about fitness. It will take you from the big picture—how fit North America is—to a more specific concern—how fit you are. You'll also see how fit law enforcement officers are compared to the rest of the population.

Chapter 1 defines total fitness and its components. It discusses why fitness is important to law enforcement officers and gives you some examples of the types of activities that require fitness. You'll read some alarming statistics about the fitness and health of North Americans and recognize that many of these problems aren't caused by germs or viruses, but rather by lifestyle choices. Next, you'll learn about the fitness and health of your fellow officers. You might be surprised to see how you compare to the public at large. You'll also hear what some law enforcement professional groups have to say about the issue. Finally, chapter 1 discusses the benefits of a fitness program. These benefits include improved performance and better health, and they help the organization as well as the individual.

Chapter 2 is aimed specifically at sedentary officers and those with low fitness levels. It provides guidelines and tips for becoming more physically active and includes a starter program to prepare you for the fitness assessments presented in chapter 3. Chapter 2 also provides some precautions to help ensure your safety. You'll learn that increasing physical activity is a step toward beginning a more structured exercise program.

Chapter 3 gives you the opportunity to assess your own fitness level. If your agency does not administer a fitness test, the simple assessments provided will help you measure your current level of physical fitness.

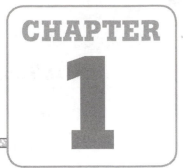

What Does Fitness Mean to an Officer?

You hear the word *fitness* often, and although you may have some idea what it means, it's used to describe several different conditions and concepts. Generally, when people hear the term, they think of physical fitness. Physical fitness is the ability to perform physical activities such as job tasks with enough reserve for emergency situations and for enjoying recreational pursuits. That is an important part of fitness, but there is more to being fit than just being able to exercise. As noted in the preface, this book is based on a concept of *total fitness,* or the ability to perform physical activities while being free of health problems. This chapter presents information about how North Americans in general, and law enforcement officers in particular, are doing in the lifestyle fitness areas of nutrition, weight management, stress management, smoking cessation, substance abuse prevention, and exercise.

Both your health and your performance are affected by your lifestyle. For example, eating correctly will lower your risk for heart disease and other health problems while providing the energy you need to pursue suspects and engage in use-of-force situations.

HISTORY OF PHYSICAL FITNESS

Before we begin a detailed discussion of the importance of fitness to law enforcement officers, it will help to understand the history of physical fitness in North America. Before the 20th century, no formal physical fitness programs existed. The exercise Americans did was part of their daily lives. If you wanted to stay warm, you chopped some wood and carried it inside. If you went to visit a neighbor, you probably walked. To put food on the table, you tended a garden and went hunting. The demands of staying alive kept people fit.

As labor-saving devices became more available, the amount of exercise Americans did in their daily lives began to decrease. World War II was a dramatic wake-up call about the deteriorating state of readiness in America. The Armed Services were shocked to find that millions of Americans drafted for service were not fit enough for combat. As a result, the first formal fitness programs in America were developed to help get those men into shape.

After the war, with even more labor-saving devices being invented, America's physical fitness declined even more. It wasn't until the 1960s that researchers such as Dr. Kenneth Cooper began identifying a relationship between higher levels of cardiovascular fitness and decreased incidences of heart disease. Although this was an important breakthrough, the fitness and health profession may have made an error of omission at this point. The profession placed so much emphasis on the health benefits of exercise that many lost sight of the connection between exercise and job performance. The consequences of that oversight are still being felt today, and many law enforcement administrators view a fitness program as a *health* initiative. We must shift the emphasis back to the paradigm that exercise and physical fitness underlie job performance. Athletes understand the importance of exercise and fitness in improving their performance.

COMPONENTS OF PHYSICAL FITNESS

As you will learn in more detail in part II, physical fitness has eight components. The first five are commonly called functional or health-related fitness because they have a direct bearing on many health risk factors; however, they are also the underlying fitness areas that determine physical performance. The last three are often called motor fitness because they have a direct bearing on movement capabilities. All eight components encompass total fitness for the job.

Functional and Health-Related Fitness

body composition—The balance between fat and lean tissue in your body. Generally, the lower your percentage of body fat, the more efficient your movement. Having an appropriate level of body fat also contributes to good appearance, which can enhance your professional image. Body composition is most accurately estimated by underwater weighing, skinfold testing, or electrical impedance. A simpler but less accurate method is to calculate the body mass index. You'll learn how to do this in chapter 3.

cardiovascular endurance (CVE)—The ability to perform activity that requires the body to combine its energy sources with oxygen. Also referred to as aerobic power, endurance, stamina, or cardiorespiratory endurance, CVE is important to law enforcement officers for activities requiring extended effort, such as pursuits and use-of-force situations lasting more than 2 minutes.

flexibility—The range of motion of part of the body around a joint. Flexibility is important for activities involving bending and reaching.

muscular endurance—The muscles' capacity to make repeated contractions without undue fatigue. Also referred to as dynamic strength, it is important in use-of-force situations, as well as for pulling, pushing, lifting, carrying, and dragging people and things.

muscular strength—The muscles' ability to generate maximum force. Also referred to as absolute strength, it is important for activities such as pushing a disabled car out of traffic and lifting people or things.

Motor Fitness

agility—The ability to make quick movements while sprinting, which is important for making changes of direction around obstacles during pursuits.

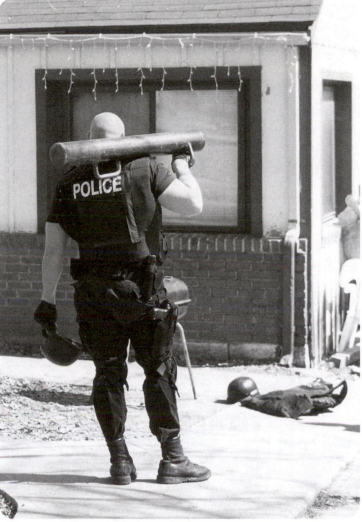

Your job encompasses many components of fitness—the functional and health-related areas and the motor fitness areas of agility, anaerobic power, and explosive power.

© Mikael Karlsson/arrestingimages.com

anaerobic power—The ability to make short, intense bursts of maximal effort, which is important in pursuit and use-of-force situations.

explosive leg strength or power—The ability to jump with power. This component also contributes to the ability to make short, intense bursts of effort and is important for performing job tasks such as jumping over obstacles and sprinting in pursuit situations.

These fitness areas (both functional and motor fitness) are the underlying physical factors (abilities) in performing the essential physical tasks of the job. Physical fitness tests (as shown on page 6 and discussed in detail in chapter 3) can measure these fitness factors. Since they are easily administered field tests, you can use them to help develop your fitness program.

Physical Fitness Factors and Tests

Fitness factor	Test
Absolute strength for the upper body	1RM bench press raw score in pounds 1RM bench press ratio score (weight pressed divided by body weight)
Explosive leg strength	Vertical jump in inches

Dynamic strength
    Abdominal muscular endurance
    Upper body muscular endurance
	
	1-minute sit-up test (number completed)
	Maximum push-up test (number completed)

Extent flexibility	Sit-and-reach test in inches
Endurance/aerobic power	1.5-mile run in min:sec or 1-mile walk test
Anaerobic power	300-meter run in seconds
Agility	Illinois agility run in seconds
Body composition	Skinfolds or body mass index (BMI)

FITNESS ON THE JOB

Fitness is important to everyone. The more fit you are, the easier it is to deal with just about every aspect of life. And if being fit can have a positive impact on your home life, just imagine what it can do for your performance on the job!

As you already know, the physical demands of your job may be infrequent, but they can be tough. In a pursuit situation, you may be running, climbing, jumping, or using force. To help protect civilians in an emergency, you may have to lift, carry, drag, pull, or push objects. And to make things even more difficult, you'll probably have to go from relative inactivity to high gear with little or no warning.

To give you an idea of the level of effort these tasks entail, here is some information that describes the physical demands on law enforcement officers. Some of this information comes from the Multijurisdictional Law Enforcement Physical Skills Survey conducted by Wollack & Associates (1992). Since 1992, we have collected physical demand data from more than 4,000 law enforcement officers representing more than 85 agencies. A review of the two sets of data shows that the job involves physical demands, and they are pretty consistent. Here is a summary of those demands.

- **Running.** The most frequent running tasks lasted less than a minute; however, more than 11 percent of running tasks took more than 2 minutes. Surmounting and avoiding obstacles were required in most running situations. Our data indicated that the average maximum pursuit distance was approximately 500 yards, with one-third of pursuits occurring over uneven terrain.

- **Climbing.** Most fences climbed were 5 feet high or less. For stairs, one or two flights were usually involved. Quickness was important for both types of climbing. Our data showed that the average fence height was 6 feet, and officers climbed four or five flights of stairs.
- **Jumping.** Vaulting and jumping were generally done over obstacles of 3 feet or less. Our sample reported jumping heights and widths between 4 and 5 feet.
- **Lifting and carrying.** The majority of lifting and carrying tasks were performed unassisted, with weights of 50 pounds or less being carried for distances of 20 feet or less. Our data indicated that the average weight lifted was approximately 65 pounds and the average carrying distance was 35 feet.
- **Dragging.** Dragging and pulling tasks were predominantly unassisted, with most objects weighing less than 100 pounds and being moved less than 10 feet. Our data suggested that the average weight was between 100 and 150 pounds and that the dragging distance was approximately 20 feet.
- **Pushing.** Most of the pushed objects weighed less than 100 pounds and were pushed a distance of less than 10 feet. Our data indicated that the average weight was between 100 and 150 pounds and the pushing distance was between 20 and 30 feet. For pushing vehicles, the 1992 data showed that the distance moved was usually more than 30 feet and the move was done in less than a minute. Our data showed similar results.
- **Use of force.** For more than 75 percent of apprehensions, the amount of resistance was moderate or strong. In most of the occurrences, immediate officer attention was required. The time it took to subdue a suspect was equally distributed among 30, 60, and 120 seconds or more. Our data suggested that the average weight of a suspect was 200 pounds.
- **Energy cost.** For many of the sustained physical tasks lasting more than 2 minutes (such as pursuits and use-of-force situations), the level of stamina required of officers was often 75 to 90 percent of their maximum capability. Our data suggested similar results.

The results from these two databases suggest that the physical demands of the job can be very high and that over the past 10 years those demands have increased. However, it appears that not all officers possess the underlying fitness to perform those physical tasks. Between 10 and 20 percent of the officers tested in our validation studies were unable to perform physical job tasks such as a running pursuit or victim extraction at a minimal level of proficiency.

Performing Essential Tasks

You may feel that because your job doesn't often require you to perform physically exerting tasks, physical fitness isn't crucial. However, you also have to consider the importance of the situations in which fitness is a factor. Many of the physical tasks associated with your job, even if not performed often, can have unfavorable consequences if you are unable to perform them adequately.

Our database of more than 4,000 officers results from more than 35 validation studies we conducted to define job-related physical fitness standards for approximately 85 federal, state, and municipal agencies. The physical demand data previously reported were collected using a job task analysis, which included ratings of frequency and criticality. Incumbent officers consistently rated 18 physical tasks as either frequent or critical:

Bending and reaching

Climbing fences

Climbing stairs

Crawling under or through obstacles

Dodging obstacles

Dragging objects

Extracting or dragging victims

Jumping over obstacles

Light, medium, and heavy lifting and carrying

Pushing heavy objects such as cars

Running over uneven terrain

Running short and long distances

Running up and down stairs

Short- and long-term use of force

Using the hands and feet in self-defense

Using restraining devices

Vaulting over obstacles

Walking

We operationalized those tasks into three job task simulation tests representing real-world job-related scenarios:

- Roadway clearance, involving lifting, carrying, and dragging debris and pushing a car
- Victim extraction, involving sprinting to a disabled vehicle and lifting and dragging a dummy to safety
- Sustained foot pursuit, involving running up stairs, dodging, jumping, climbing a fence, crawling, vaulting obstacles, striking and moving a dummy, and simulated handcuffing using resistance bands

Of the officers tested in the validation studies, 95 percent stated that they had either experienced or would expect to encounter those scenarios. This further clarifies the physical nature of the job.

Another study considered how often each of 20 physical tasks was performed annually, both in absolute numbers and as percentages of workdays in a year. The percentages ranged from 1 to 32 percent, so you might think the tasks weren't performed often enough to worry about. However, when the officers participating in our 35 validation studies rated the consequences of inadequate performance of the tasks contained in the three job task simulations, we again found that criticality is considered more important than frequency. For each scenario, officers selected one or more of the following as possible consequences of inability to perform the task. Here are the results:

66 percent	Failure to provide needed service
30 percent	Property loss or damage
66 percent	Failure to apprehend suspect
70 percent	Possible injury risk
65 percent	Possible loss of life

Further analysis of the 35 validation studies defined the primary and secondary fitness factors for performing frequent and critical law enforcement physical tasks (see below).

Body composition was not a primary or secondary factor. One reason is that cardiovascular endurance, strength, and muscular endurance are all related to body composition. As long as those fitness areas are measured, the effect of body fat is not as noticeable. The key is having the fitness capabilities to perform strenuous activities.

Primary and Secondary Fitness Factors

Tasks	Primary fitness	Secondary fitness
Sustained pursuit	Cardiovascular endurance	Muscular endurance Agility
Short sprints	Anaerobic power	Explosive leg power
Lifting and carrying	Upper body strength	Muscular endurance Explosive leg power
Jumping and vaulting	Explosive leg power	Anaerobic power
Climbing stairs and fences	Anaerobic power	Muscular endurance Agility
Dragging and pulling	Upper body strength	Muscular endurance Explosive leg power
Pushing	Upper body strength	Explosive leg power
Dodging obstacles	Agility	Anaerobic power
Bending and reaching	Flexibility	
Use-of-force situation lasting less than 2 minutes	Anaerobic power	Muscular strength Muscular endurance Agility
Use-of-force situation lasting more than 2 minutes	Cardiovascular endurance	Muscular strength Muscular endurance Agility

Note: All tasks may require some cardiovascular endurance, depending on the situation.

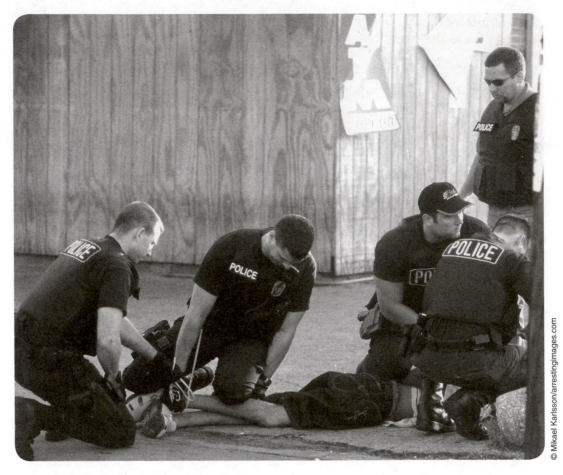

If you're physically unable to do your job effectively, you're jeopardizing not only yourself but the people you serve as well.

The bottom line is that it doesn't matter how infrequently you may be called on to perform a physical task if it is critical. If you're not fit enough, at best, you've failed in your duty; at worst, you or someone else may be killed. It's the same as needing to maintain firearm skills. You may rarely use your weapon, but when shooting skill is needed, it's critical that you have it. Likewise, if you do not have the underlying abilities (good eyesight, a steady hand for firearms proficiency, or the primary and secondary fitness factors for performing physical tasks), you may be unable to perform a critical job function.

Maintaining a Professional Image

Part of an officer's effectiveness within the community is based on the image the officer presents. The public judges officers by their physical appearance and their lifestyle, both of which are related to fitness. The judgment affects how well "police presence" can have a deterrent effect.

A national organization has analyzed case studies of officers who were severely beaten during attempted arrests. Virtually every one of the assailants said they "wanted to hurt the officer" because it was readily apparent that the officers lacked the physical wherewithal to defend themselves. This "offended" the assailants. Fitness as a means of improving an officer's image also reflects the recent trend toward improving the professionalism of law enforcement officials. Agencies have focused on areas such as officers' ethics, cognitive functioning, and interpersonal and social skills; they should also include fitness in their initiatives.

There has always been general consensus that law enforcement officers require some level of physical fitness. However, a disturbing opinion is being expressed that modern-day law enforcement requires little physical effort and, as a consequence, fitness standards or programs are not necessary. For example, some officers argue that good interpersonal and verbal skills can diffuse many potential use-of-force situations. Although that may be true at a general level, the critical incident reports we have reviewed suggest otherwise. In turn, the data we have amassed from numerous job task analyses clearly show that the job entails both frequent and critical physical demands. Much of this false perception of the physical nature of the job has emerged out of a concern for diversity and a lack of full inclusion of women within the field. Although the need to expand opportunities for women is valid, it should not be met at the expense of reduced job-related performance capabilities.

By now, the link between an officer's fitness and job performance should be clear. That's half of the total fitness definition—the capability to perform physical tasks. The other half is an officer's health. To get the big picture, let's start with Americans' fitness and health in general, then see how law enforcement officers fare compared to the general population.

SOCIETY'S FITNESS AND HEALTH

The Office of Health Promotion and Disease Prevention of the U.S. Department of Health and Human Services publishes a report every 10 years with health statistics and defined health goals for the nation. The most recent report, *Healthy People 2010*, rates physical activity and fitness as the primary focus area for national health goals (USDHHS 2000). Americans generally are not as fit as they should be. This lack of fitness can mean more than poor job performance—it can lead to disability or death. The Public Health Agency of Canada likewise periodically publishes health and fitness findings. Following are the most recent statistics from both Canada and the United States.

- In 2001, cardiovascular (heart) diseases killed more than 700,000 Americans (approximately 30 percent of all deaths). Although this rate is less than half of what it was in 1967 due to efforts aimed at smoking cessation and lowering cholesterol, as well as better medical care, it is still largely due to lifestyle choices. Thus, there is room for even more improvement. Cardiovascular disease is also the number-one killer in Canada. In 2001, 33 percent of male and 35 percent of female deaths were due to cardiovascular disease.

- In 2001, an estimated 538,000 Americans—almost 1,500 a day—died of cancer. One of every four deaths in the United States is due to cancer, predominantly lung and breast cancers. The incidence of cancer deaths in Canada is even higher: 37 percent in 2002. That year, 136,900 new cases were reported along with 66,200 deaths.

- In 2002, 420,000 Americans died of diseases related to tobacco use. About 85 percent of lung cancer cases in the United States are due to cigarette smoking. In Canada, tobacco use is the cause of 30 percent of all cancers and contributes to approximately 45,000 deaths per year.

- The Centers for Disease Control and Prevention (CDC), the agency responsible for disease prevention in the United States, estimates that by 2006, poor nutrition and a sedentary lifestyle will overtake tobacco as the leading cause of death in America. The Public Health Agency of Canada estimates that 20 percent of all cancers in that country are related to poor nutrition.

- Some 21 percent of all Americans are being treated for high cholesterol. No cholesterol studies have been conducted in Canada for the past 10 years, but the problem is likely similar there as well.

- About 64 percent of Americans are overweight, with 31 percent being obese. Of significance is that between 1997 and 2000, obesity has increased by 35 percent in the United States and the number of overweight Americans has increased by 14 percent. Obesity among teenage boys in Canada has increased from 16 to 22 percent in the past 15 years, and the percentage of obese girls has doubled during the same time period.

- Between 1997 and 2000, the incidence of diabetes has increased 16 percent within the U.S. population. Experts estimate that 64 percent of Americans over age 20 who are diagnosed with diabetes are obese or overweight.

- Some 17 million Americans and 2.25 million Canadians have adult-onset diabetes. It is the seventh-leading cause of death in Canada, with 60,000 new cases reported each year.

- Although 80 percent of people with osteoporosis are women, 2 million men suffer from this condition, with 12 million more at risk. The Public Health Agency of Canada estimates that one of every four women and one of every eight men over 50 have osteoporosis.

- Americans have an 8-in-10 chance of experiencing back pain sometime in their adult lives; 18 percent of the Canadian population seeks medical attention for back pain each year.

- Some 28 percent of Americans and 22 percent of Canadians are being treated for high blood pressure, a major risk factor for stroke. An estimated 140,000 deaths a year are due to stroke, the third major cause of death.

- In the United States, about two-thirds of all visits to primary-care physicians are stress related, 112 million people take medication for stress, and industry loses more than $150 billion annually due to stress-related problems.

- During 1998, the cost of alcohol-abuse problems in the United States was estimated at $184.6 billion, a 25 percent increase from 1990. Ten percent of Canadians consider themselves to be heavy drinkers.

- In 2000, the cost of drug abuse in the United States was $160.7 billion.

- Experts estimate that hundreds of thousands of Americans abuse anabolic steroids. In 1997, about 175,000 teenage girls reported taking steroids, an increase of more than 100 percent since 1991. The rate among teenage boys has continued to rise to the current estimated level of 325,000.

- About 28 percent of Americans and 16 percent of Canadians report activity limitations due to orthopedic and arthritic conditions.

- One in five adults have mental health problems, and recent data indicate a link between depression and heart disease.

- Total health expenditures for Canadians in 2001 were $97.6 billion, up 7.2 percent from the previous year. That represents an average of $3,174 per person.

These statistics are staggering, but if you believe that "forewarned is forearmed," you need to know about them. These conditions are not communicable illnesses caused by viruses or bacteria; they are related to poor fitness. The lifestyle choices you make—how you eat, whether you exercise, how you deal with stress—and many other factors in your daily life influence whether you develop them. The good news about these medical problems is that you can do something to combat them. The major causes of death and disability are well documented and include sedentary living, poor nutrition, obesity, stress, tobacco smoking, and substance abuse.

Sedentary Living   Only 20 percent of Americans exercise vigorously three times a week. Approximately 40 percent do some type of moderate activity, and 40 percent are completely sedentary. Some 300,000 premature deaths are due to sedentary lifestyles, with a health care cost of more than $90 billion. Studies show that sedentary people run twice the risk of coronary heart disease than active people do. They also have a higher risk for stroke and colon cancer and may be more prone to back injury and stress-related problems. In addition, there is growing evidence that lack of exercise is a risk factor for certain mental health conditions such as depression and anxiety. The CDC is recognizing inactivity as one of the top two health problems facing the nation.

Poor Nutrition   The typical American diet is too high in calories (leading to the obesity epidemic), with dietary fat currently making up 36 percent of the calories consumed. Too much dietary fat can create a higher risk of heart disease, breast and colon cancer, and possibly gallbladder disease. Too little fiber can create a risk of colon cancer or diverticulosis; too little calcium can lead to osteoporosis and may be related to colon cancer and high blood pressure. The latest surveys also indicate that only 28 percent of Americans get the recommended servings of fruit, 3 percent of Americans get the recommended servings of vegetables, and 7 percent of Americans get the recommended servings of grains.

Obesity   About two-thirds of American adults are overweight, with a third of them being obese; that is, they have unhealthy amounts of body fat. Obesity has been linked to many chronic diseases such as diabetes, hypertension, and cancer. About 65 percent of the diseases Americans die from are related to obesity, and it may also exacerbate orthopedic and lower back problems. Many researchers consider obesity as deadly as smoking.

Stress   We all have stress in our lives, but the ability to control stress affects our health and fitness. Stress can be a secondary risk factor in major health problems such as heart disease, hypertension, cancer, ulcers, and low back pain.

Smoking   More than 50 million Americans smoke. Tobacco smoking doubles the risk of heart attacks, causes 20 percent of deaths due to stroke and 85 percent of those due to lung cancer, and is linked to other types of cancer, emphysema, and chronic bronchitis. Recent research seems to indicate that secondhand smoke causes health problems for nonsmokers. Some studies even estimate that secondhand smoke leads to 47,000 deaths per year. Researchers also suspect a yet-unexplained connection between smoking and low back pain. Despite some recent reduction in the number of smokers, smoking is still responsible for one of every six deaths in the United States, or about 400,000 annually.

Substance Abuse   Approximately 18 million Americans currently have problems due to alcohol, and about 7 percent of alcohol drinkers exhibit moderate levels of dependency symptoms. Alcohol abuse can damage brain cells, the liver, and other vital organs. It also increases the risk of cancer, heart disease, high blood pressure, and nervous disorders. Substance abuse of any kind can lead to violence or accidents.

These statistics have led to international and national efforts to educate the public about the need for lifestyle change. The *Healthy People 2010* report set specific national goals for increasing physical activity and exercise, preventing obesity, improving nutritional habits, decreasing smoking and substance abuse, and addressing mental health problems (USDHHS 2000). The *Report on Physical Activity and Health* issued by the Surgeon General of the U.S. Public Health Service in 1996 identified inactivity as the major risk factor for disease in the 21st century and recommended exercise (leading to physical fitness) as the major lifestyle element to incorporate into daily living to prevent disease and premature death. Even the World Health Organization (WHO) is recognizing inactivity as a major worldwide health problem (USDHHS 1996).

Clearly, many Americans are not fit and pay for it with poor health. How do law enforcement officers measure up to the general population?

OFFICERS' FITNESS AND HEALTH

Although no national databases allow for a comprehensive assessment of fitness levels, The Cooper Institute in Dallas, Texas, has been measuring the physical performance of various populations for some years. Their data on more than 30,000 subjects are often used as a reference when evaluating physical performance. Let's consider some studies that compare law enforcement performance against these data.

The first attempt to draw inferences about officer fitness was a study conducted by the International Association of Chiefs of Police (1977). For a sample of 203 officers, cardiorespiratory endurance levels and percent body fat approached only the 25th percentile of the general population (75 percent of the general population scored better). Upper body and abdominal strength were between the 20th and 35th percentiles, and flexibility scores were at the 45th percentile. These figures suggest that the officers studied were fatter, weaker, and had less stamina and flexibility than the general population they were responsible for safeguarding.

One of the populations The Cooper Institute has studied is the law enforcement profession. From 1983 to 1990, they found some improvement in baseline fitness. Officers' aerobic fitness approached the 35th percentile of the general population, with body fat at the 30th percentile. Upper body strength and flexibility were approximately at the 50th percentile, with abdominal strength at the 40th percentile.

The 1992 Penn State Aging Study collected data for 5,000 to 10,000 officers in six large agencies (Landy 1992). The results of this survey suggest that officers are below average in aerobic fitness and body fat but somewhat above average in strength and lower back flexibility.

The most recent data from our validation studies, conducted since 1992, include test results for more than 4,000 officers. The data indicate that fitness levels for younger male officers are average or above average for all areas compared to the general population. One reason may be that the general population (especially adolescents and young adults) as a whole is less fit due to decreased physical activity. As a consequence, younger officers who have recently undergone basic academy training score at higher levels on fitness tests. Older officers tend to score at or below average. Special units such as SWAT teams had the highest fitness levels.

These data suggest two things. First, even younger officers are at best only as fit as their civilian contemporaries. Second, they compare even less favorably the longer they are on the force. Why is this?

One reason is that their jobs entail little day-to-day physical activity. Unlike a lumberjack, for example, whose work keeps him fit, an officer must develop physical fitness off the job. In addition, irregular hours and unpredictable meal schedules can contribute to poor nutrition. Finally, several aspects of the job contribute to stress: the potential danger, the need to switch quickly from inaction to action, dealing with people who are upset or angry, or even inactivity itself. Many choose to deal with these stressors by overeating, smoking, or abusing alcohol. All of these factors taken together can create a vicious cycle from which it becomes difficult to escape. These lifestyle choices affect not only performance but health as well.

It is impossible to discuss fitness without mentioning its health implications. Research findings have consistently shown a link between lifestyle and disease. What you eat, whether you smoke, how much alcohol you consume, how you deal with stress, and your physical fitness all have a direct bearing on your health as well as your job performance.

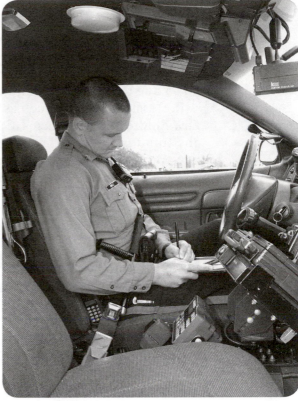

Sitting in a patrol car does nothing to improve fitness. Finding ways to be physically active outside of work is necessary for good health.

Mortality statistics suggest that law enforcement officers are at increased risk for premature death and may be especially vulnerable to certain diseases. Most studies indicate that law enforcement officers die at earlier ages than expected for the general population for all causes of death and in particular for diabetes, colon cancer, and cardiovascular disease. Studies also show that law enforcement officers have a higher suicide rate than the general population. This may be due to the amount of stress associated with the work.

The Cooper studies examined the medical histories of law enforcement officers employed in small, medium, and large local, state, and federal agencies. The resulting data showed the percentages of incumbents who had major medical problems:

Medical or health condition	Officers with condition
Obesity	20 to 50 percent
Heart disease	5 to 10 percent
High cholesterol	20 to 30 percent
Back and orthopedic problems	15 to 25 percent
Psychological problems	8 to 25 percent
Hypertension	4 to 15 percent

Survey data indicate that only 80 percent of officers reach scheduled retirement; 14 percent take early retirement due to medical problems and 6 percent die while employed as law enforcement officers. Even among the retired officers, a large percentage are in some sort of disability status. For example, the California Peace Officers' Association reports that 73 percent of all officers who retire in that state do so due to a disability (*Law and Order* 1994).

Professional groups such as the IACP and the Commission on Accreditation for Law Enforcement Agencies (CALEA), as well as many state peace officer standards and training councils, have recognized that fitness and health problems exist and have proposed policies in an attempt to alleviate their effects. The International Association of State Directors of Law Enforcement Training recently recommended that physical fitness standards and programs be initiated in all law enforcement agencies.

BENEFITS OF A FITNESS PROGRAM

So far, we've discussed some of the negative effects of lack of fitness. Here are some of the personal benefits of an effective fitness program.

Better Job Performance

Studies have found that more physically fit officers generally receive higher job performance ratings. Some additional job performance benefits are as follows.

- **Improved performance of essential physical tasks.** For the unfit, this improvement may equate to satisfactory performance in areas that were previously below par. For the already fit, it may mean improving satisfactory performance to an even higher level.

- **Reduced likelihood of using excessive force.** Fitter, more confident officers are less likely to be involved in use-of-force situations for several reasons. A suspect may think twice about challenging a physically fit officer. Conversely, a physically fit officer may be able to meet a physical challenge without resorting to the next level of force; for example, going from grappling to using a baton. Finally, a physically fit officer is likely to overcome a suspect on foot and avoid having to use more force than necessary to prevent someone from fleeing the scene.

Improved Health

In addition to improved performance, you are likely to see the following health benefits.

- **Prevention of health problems.** Increased fitness not only restores health but also prevents health problems from developing. For example, regular vigorous physical activity helps prevent coronary heart disease and assists in weight control. Exercise that builds muscular strength and endurance and develops flexibility may protect against injury, disability, and osteoporosis. Physical activity also can bring about changes that help prevent and control hypertension (high blood pressure), heart disease, and diabetes.

- **Longer life.** Increased fitness can also contribute to longevity. In a study of 16,936 Harvard alumni over a 16-year period, those who expended at least 2,000 calories per week in physical activity had a 28 percent lower risk of death from any cause (Paffenbarger et al. 1986).

- **Better quality of life.** Increased fitness can improve people's daily lives. Participants in fitness programs have less fatigue and greater productivity. Regular exercise has also been shown to help reduce anxiety and tension and reduce cardiovascular reactions to stress. And the latest research is demonstrating that fitness can help prevent depression and anxiety and increase self-esteem.

- **Less risk of disability.** You've worked hard at your profession and certainly look forward to a well-deserved retirement. The numbers show that many of your colleagues are unable to enjoy their retirement years fully because of health problems that are directly related to lifestyle choices. Making changes in your lifestyle now can help ensure that you get to enjoy what you have worked so hard for.

Lower Department Costs

The following benefits are common among workers involved in a fitness program.

- **Fewer sick days.** Fit and active employees have lower absenteeism rates. Companies report 20 to 35 percent reductions in absenteeism after the initiation of a worksite fitness program. Studies performed with law enforcement officers indicate that the more fit and active officers, especially those over age 35, have lower absenteeism rates. One agency reported an 87 percent drop in sick time due to job-related injuries. Another found that officers using the fitness center more than 50 times a year used seven fewer sick days per year than those using the center fewer than 50 times a year.

- **Improved productivity.** Fitness and productivity tend to be positively related. Data from occupations such as salespeople, textile workers, and office workers indicate that active workers have higher productivity. Studies of law enforcement officers that analyzed their supervisors' ratings of performance indicated that the more fit and active officers obtained higher ratings.

- **Reduced health care costs.** Preliminary data suggest that the introduction of a worksite fitness program reduces worker health care costs. Several studies found that medical expenses dropped for participating and active employees. A risk manager analyzing statewide health care costs found that fit and unfit officers suffered about the same number of on-duty injuries. However, the fit officers tended to get hurt while making arrests and conducting foot pursuits. The unfit officers' injuries were more mundane, such as turning ankles while stepping off curbs. Moreover, although the number of injuries for the two groups was the same, the unfit officers cost the state 10 times more money! Having higher levels of fitness helped officers get back to work more quickly. Lower agency health care costs mean more money for your agency to spend in other areas, such as training programs, salaries, and benefits.

What do all these statistics add up to? The data presented make a case for the necessity of being fit for the job and for your health. The numbers are overwhelming because they reflect the consequences of poor lifestyle choices. Addressing your physical fitness is ultimately a personal choice. You may sense that you are not at the top of your game or wish you had more energy or just want to look good. You may want to have the energy to be more active with the kids or to enjoy your retirement.

For any of these reasons, some of you might recognize that you need to do something about your fitness. Others of you may feel that your fitness level is adequate. Still others of you may not have a clue as to your status. For those who need it, chapter 2 will give you some ideas on getting started. Others may choose to skip ahead to chapter 3, which will help you assess your status in several fitness areas. Both chapters will help you determine a starting point for your new lifestyle.

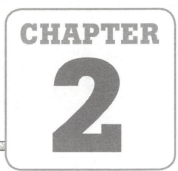

How Do You Get Started?

Presumably, the previous chapter's discussion of the rationale for becoming more fit has helped you understand the need to be active. The next step is to act on that understanding. This chapter provides guidelines and tips for getting started on an activity program. The first step toward becoming more physically active is to incorporate daily movement into your life. The goal is for daily physical activity to eventually lead to a more formal physical exercise program. Depending on your current level of activity, you may find a starter program helpful. You'll find one at the end of this chapter.

For many who have been sedentary, the notion of getting dressed in workout clothes and going to a gym to exercise is just too much of a behavioral change. So you may have to start by trying to incorporate physical activity into your daily life as an intermediate step before engaging in more fitness-related physical activities. Initiating a starter program can help you develop the physical activity habit gradually. Once you have the habit, following a more strenuous exercise program on a sustained basis becomes easier. If you don't get much physical activity or exercise and are basically sedentary, this chapter is an important transition to a full-scale fitness program. For those who perform at least 30 minutes of physical activity on a daily basis, you can skip this chapter or use it as a review.

EXERCISE VERSUS PHYSICAL ACTIVITY

In differentiating between an exercise program and a physical activity program, we first have to look at the goals of each. The goals of a planned, structured, systematic, and repetitive exercise program are to increase physical fitness and physical performance capacity. The goal of a physical activity program is to incorporate

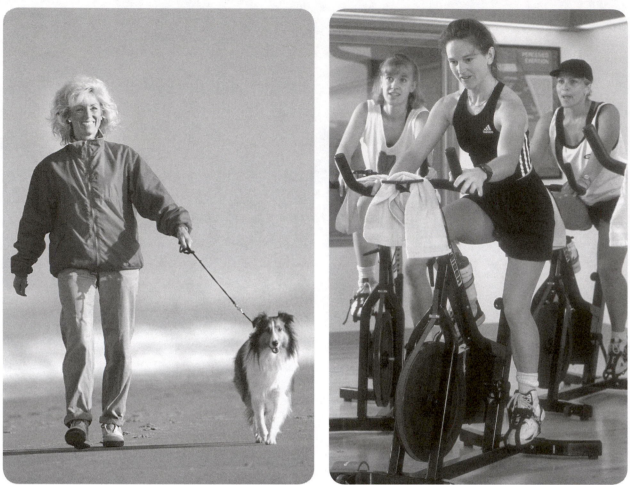

A physical activity program is about incorporating some informal movement into your day. An exercise program is about structured movement.

movement into your daily life so that it becomes a habit. It is not as structured or intense as the exercise program you will design later. It is simply about adding more physical movement to your life.

Both physical activity and exercise involve the expenditure of energy. For the human body, we define energy in terms of calories. The body takes in calories (in the form of food) that serve as the fuel for sustaining necessary bodily functions (metabolism). The body at rest burns fewer calories than it does during activity. The more activity the body performs, the more calories are utilized. Both physical activity and exercise are movements that burn calories. Structured, repetitive exercise is more intense, burning more calories per minute; however, the body will burn more calories per minute even during less intense activity than it burns at rest. You can equalize calorie utilization by performing less intense activity for a longer duration.

Light and moderate physical activities include leisure walking, gardening, and housework. More intense activities that burn more calories include jogging, weight training, tennis, and soccer. The energy cost (expressed as calories per minute) will vary depending on body weight. For the same activities, heavier people burn more calories per minute. The calorie costs of sample activities for a 150-pound person are shown in the box to the right.

The important thing is that you are moving your body to burn more calories. The processes of activity and exercise stimulate the body to make changes, resulting in greater stamina, more strength, reduced risk to health, and better control of body weight.

The rest of this chapter presents a process to help you develop the physical activity habit that consists of four phases:

- Readiness
- Commitment
- Initiation
- Follow-through

Calorie Costs

Activity	Calorie costs
Sitting	1.3 cal/min
Standing	1.5 cal/min
Making a bed	3.4 cal/min
Dancing	5.0 cal/min
Gardening	5.6 cal/min
Walking (3.5 mph)	7.0 cal/min
Climbing stairs	8.5 cal/min
Tennis	9.0 cal/min
Running (7.5 mph)	15.0 cal/min

PREPARING FOR ACTIVITY

The first phase is getting ready to be active. At this point, you understand the benefits of being active. Now it's time to develop a personal reason for becoming more physically active. You may decide to get ready for one or more of the following reasons:

- Emotional: combat depression
- Mental: improve alertness
- Physical: lose weight
- Health: prevent heart disease
- Performance: be someone your partner can count on

You are more likely to be successful in adopting a new habit if you have a sense of why it is important to you.

Weighing the Activity Choice

You are also more likely to make this change if the benefits of being active outweigh the perceived difficulties or negative aspects of physical activity. One way to help assess the value of becoming physically active is to weigh the reasons for and against starting a program. Common advantages and disadvantages that might be identified when you weigh the benefits of starting an activity program are shown on the following page. Spaces are provided at the end of the list for you to add your personal pros and cons.

Choosing to start an activity program is a conscious decision. Being aware of these potential advantages and disadvantages can foster an informed willingness to get started. The hope is that when you compare the pros and cons, you'll find that the benefits outweigh the difficulties. This process also helps you anticipate potential problems that may influence your ability to stick with a program once you start.

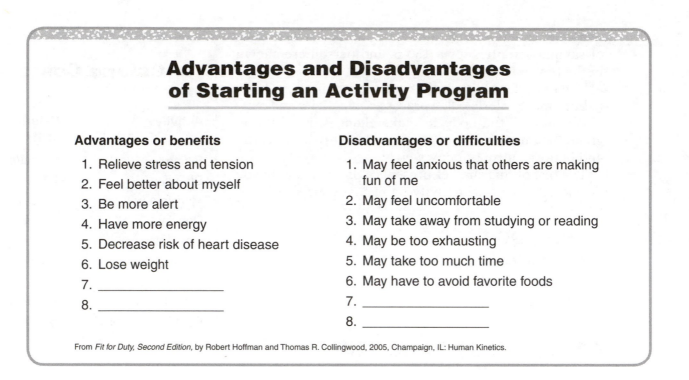

Advantages and Disadvantages of Starting an Activity Program

Advantages or benefits

1. Relieve stress and tension
2. Feel better about myself
3. Be more alert
4. Have more energy
5. Decrease risk of heart disease
6. Lose weight
7. _____
8. _____

Disadvantages or difficulties

1. May feel anxious that others are making fun of me
2. May feel uncomfortable
3. May take away from studying or reading
4. May be too exhausting
5. May take too much time
6. May have to avoid favorite foods
7. _____
8. _____

From *Fit for Duty, Second Edition,* by Robert Hoffman and Thomas R. Collingwood, 2005, Champaign, IL: Human Kinetics.

Determining Physical Readiness

Another key step in getting ready is to determine if it is safe for you to engage in physical activity. Individuals who are apparently healthy can usually participate in mild or moderate exercise (such as walking) without any problems and without the need for a medical examination. However, strenuous or even moderate exercise can be risky for people with certain health problems. That's why it is essential that you undergo screening for such health problems before you begin fitness testing and an exercise program. Screening can help identify whether you are likely to have a problem and thus need to see a doctor before you begin.

A self-administered screening tool, Par-Q & You (see the following page), includes a preparticipation checklist that will help you identify whether you should consult a doctor before beginning an activity program. Answer each question yes or no. If you answer yes to any questions, you should call or visit your doctor before beginning an activity program. The Par-Q (Physical Activity Readiness Questionnaire) is a good screening tool and easy to administer, but there are other indicators of your relative risk for exercise. The following information is included for those whose concerns about their risk for exercise persist after reviewing the Par-Q. These tests provide information to help determine your readiness and result in baseline measurements you can use to monitor your progress throughout your training program.

- **Height.** Take this measurement in your stocking feet. Your fitness program won't change your height, but you'll use this measurement later to determine your body mass index, an estimate of how much body fat you have.
- **Weight.** Weigh yourself wearing as little clothing as you are comfortable with, and try to dress the same for subsequent weighings.
- **Resting heart rate (RHR).** Sit quietly for at least 5 minutes before taking this measurement. You will need a stopwatch or a watch with a sweep second hand. Locate your pulse in one of two places: your carotid pulse, located at

Physical Activity Readiness
Questionnaire - PAR-Q
(revised 2002)

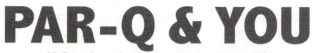

PAR-Q & YOU

(A Questionnaire for People Aged 15 to 69)

Regular physical activity is fun and healthy, and increasingly more people are starting to become more active every day. Being more active is very safe for most people. However, some people should check with their doctor before they start becoming much more physically active.

If you are planning to become much more physically active than you are now, start by answering the seven questions in the box below. If you are between the ages of 15 and 69, the PAR-Q will tell you if you should check with your doctor before you start. If you are over 69 years of age, and you are not used to being very active, check with your doctor.

Common sense is your best guide when you answer these questions. Please read the questions carefully and answer each one honestly: check YES or NO.

YES	NO		
☐	☐	1.	**Has your doctor ever said that you have a heart condition <u>and</u> that you should only do physical activity recommended by a doctor?**
☐	☐	2.	**Do you feel pain in your chest when you do physical activity?**
☐	☐	3.	**In the past month, have you had chest pain when you were not doing physical activity?**
☐	☐	4.	**Do you lose your balance because of dizziness or do you ever lose consciousness?**
☐	☐	5.	**Do you have a bone or joint problem (for example, back, knee or hip) that could be made worse by a change in your physical activity?**
☐	☐	6.	**Is your doctor currently prescribing drugs (for example, water pills) for your blood pressure or heart condition?**
☐	☐	7.	**Do you know of <u>any other reason</u> why you should not do physical activity?**

If

you

answered

YES to one or more questions

Talk with your doctor by phone or in person BEFORE you start becoming much more physically active or BEFORE you have a fitness appraisal. Tell your doctor about the PAR-Q and which questions you answered YES.

- You may be able to do any activity you want — as long as you start slowly and build up gradually. Or, you may need to restrict your activities to those which are safe for you. Talk with your doctor about the kinds of activities you wish to participate in and follow his/her advice.
- Find out which community programs are safe and helpful for you.

NO to all questions

If you answered NO honestly to <u>all</u> PAR-Q questions, you can be reasonably sure that you can:
- start becoming much more physically active — begin slowly and build up gradually. This is the safest and easiest way to go.
- take part in a fitness appraisal — this is an excellent way to determine your basic fitness so that you can plan the best way for you to live actively. It is also highly recommended that you have your blood pressure evaluated. If your reading is over 144/94, talk with your doctor before you start becoming much more physically active.

DELAY BECOMING MUCH MORE ACTIVE:
- if you are not feeling well because of a temporary illness such as a cold or a fever — wait until you feel better; or
- if you are or may be pregnant — talk to your doctor before you start becoming more active.

PLEASE NOTE: If your health changes so that you then answer YES to any of the above questions, tell your fitness or health professional. Ask whether you should change your physical activity plan.

<u>Informed Use of the PAR-Q</u>: The Canadian Society for Exercise Physiology, Health Canada, and their agents assume no liability for persons who undertake physical activity, and if in doubt after completing this questionnaire, consult your doctor prior to physical activity.

No changes permitted. You are encouraged to photocopy the PAR-Q but only if you use the entire form.

NOTE: If the PAR-Q is being given to a person before he or she participates in a physical activity program or a fitness appraisal, this section may be used for legal or administrative purposes.

"I have read, understood and completed this questionnaire. Any questions I had were answered to my full satisfaction."

NAME _____

SIGNATURE _____   DATE _____

SIGNATURE OF PARENT _____   WITNESS _____
or GUARDIAN (for participants under the age of majority)

Note: This physical activity clearance is valid for a maximum of 12 months from the date it is completed and becomes invalid if your condition changes so that you would answer YES to any of the seven questions.

CSEP / SCPE © Canadian Society for Exercise Physiology   Supported by: 🍁 Health Canada   Santé Canada

From Physical Activity Readiness Questionnaire (PAR-Q) © 2002. Reprinted with permission from the Canadian Society for Exercise Physiology. www.csep.ca/forms.asp.

the side of your throat, or your radial pulse, located off the centerline on the thumb side of your wrist (figure 2.1). Don't use your thumb to take your pulse because it has a pulse of its own, which will confuse your count. Start your count on a beat with zero and continue for 60 seconds.

- **Resting blood pressure.** If you can get someone to take your resting blood pressure, it is useful information. Many drugstores have machines that measure blood pressure. As a minimum, you'll want to compare it with the American College of Sports Medicine (ACSM) guideline for exercise participation of 140/90.

- **Cholesterol screening.** Your agency may offer cholesterol screening. If not, local outpatient clinics and public health agencies often provide this service.

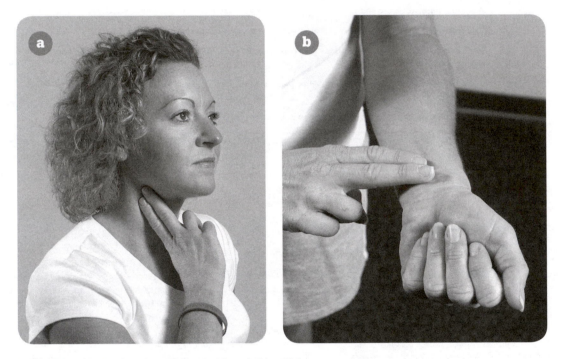

FIGURE 2.1   Pulse locations: *(a)* carotid and *(b)* radial.

Although no set of guidelines or screening method can cover every possible scenario, the ACSM has studied this matter in detail and has identified three classifications for individuals considering either exercise testing or increasing their level of physical activity.

- **Low risk.** Those who have no symptoms or complaints, appear to be healthy, and have no more than one of the major coronary risk factors listed on the top of the following page.

- **Moderate risk.** Those who have two or more major coronary risk factors or symptoms suggestive of possible cardiopulmonary (heart and lung) or metabolic disease (listed on the middle of the following page). Metabolic disease includes diabetes mellitus, thyroid disorders, renal disease, and liver disease. Men over age 45 and women over 55 are considered to have one risk factor.

- **High risk.** Those with known cardiac, pulmonary, or metabolic disease or with major signs or symptoms of those diseases.

Major Coronary Risk Factors

1. Diagnosed hypertension or systolic blood pressure ≥140 mmHg or diastolic blood pressure ≥90 mmHg on at least two separate occasions or currently on antihypertension medication
2. Total serum cholesterol ≥200 mg/dl or high-density lipoprotein cholesterol <35 mg/dl or low-density lipoprotein cholesterol >100 mg/dl
3. Cigarette smoking
4. Obesity with a body mass index >30 kg/m^2
5. Family history of coronary or other atherosclerotic disease in parents or siblings prior to age 55
6. Impaired fasting glucose >110 mg/dl
7. Sedentary lifestyle

Adapted, by permission, from American College of Sports Medicine, 2000, *ACSM's guidelines for exercise testing and prescription,* 6th ed. (Philadelphia, PA: Lippincott, Williams, and Wilkins), 25.

Major Signs Suggestive of Cardiopulmonary or Metabolic Disease

1. Pain or discomfort in the chest or surrounding areas
2. Unaccustomed shortness of breath or shortness of breath with mild exertion
3. Dizziness or faintness
4. Difficulty in breathing
5. Ankle swelling
6. Raised heart rate
7. Swelling in the lower legs
8. Known heart murmur
9. Unusual fatigue

Adapted, by permission, from American College of Sports Medicine, 2000, *ACSM's guidelines for exercise testing and prescription,* 6th ed. (Philadelphia, PA: Lippincott, Williams, and Wilkins), 24.

The ACSM recommends an examination such as a treadmill test for all people over age 45 before starting a vigorous exercise program and for higher-risk individuals of any age. For those without symptoms, this testing may not be necessary if moderate exercise is undertaken gradually with appropriate guidance and no competitive participation.

The ACSM recommends a thorough medical evaluation for all individuals with known cardiovascular, pulmonary, or metabolic disease. Determining whether it is safe to do vigorous exercise is important and provides a baseline for monitoring progress.

MAKING THE COMMITMENT

Now that you have determined you are ready for increased physical activity, the next phase is to make the commitment. This phase is the bridge between thinking about it and doing it. It involves assessing your current activity level, setting goals, and neutralizing potential barriers to increasing your activity.

Assessing Activity Level

The first step is to assess your current level of physical activity. Answering the questions below can give you an idea of your physical activity level.

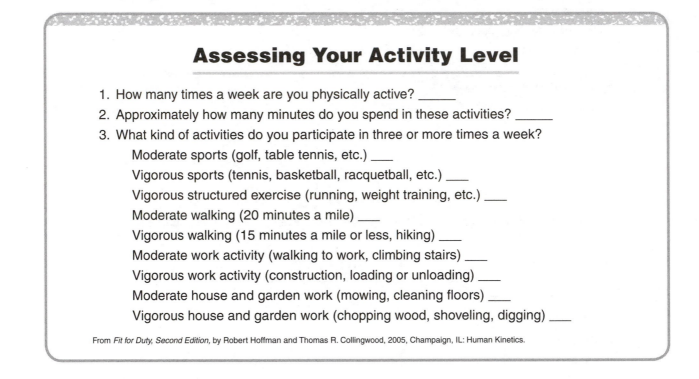

Assessing Your Activity Level

1. How many times a week are you physically active? _____
2. Approximately how many minutes do you spend in these activities? _____
3. What kind of activities do you participate in three or more times a week?
    Moderate sports (golf, table tennis, etc.) ____
    Vigorous sports (tennis, basketball, racquetball, etc.) ____
    Vigorous structured exercise (running, weight training, etc.) ____
    Moderate walking (20 minutes a mile) ____
    Vigorous walking (15 minutes a mile or less, hiking) ____
    Moderate work activity (walking to work, climbing stairs) ____
    Vigorous work activity (construction, loading or unloading) ____
    Moderate house and garden work (mowing, cleaning floors) ____
    Vigorous house and garden work (chopping wood, shoveling, digging) ____

From *Fit for Duty, Second Edition,* by Robert Hoffman and Thomas R. Collingwood, 2005, Champaign, IL: Human Kinetics.

Generally, we define "physically active" as being moderately physically active for at least 30 minutes each day of the week or exercising vigorously for at least 30 minutes three or more days a week. The type of activity can take several forms.

Setting Goals

The second step is to define your general goals for becoming more physically active. (These goals pertain to increasing activity level and are different from the fitness goals you will be setting in chapter 14.) Listing your goals for an activity program helps reinforce your effort and serves as a check for reviewing progress. These goals will likely flow from your reasons for considering an activity program. Some examples are given on the following page, with space to write down your goals. You don't need to have a goal for each area; however, the more your goals relate to your total well-being, the more likely you will be to stick with your program.

General Activity Goals

Four activity goals are defined below, followed by a sample goal. In the space provided, write your own goal for each area.

1. Emotional goals refer to how activity can aid in building a sense of self-worth and emotional stability.

Example: I will use gardening as a way to relax.

My emotional goal is _____.

2. Mental goals refer to how activity can assist mental processing.

Example: I will walk several flights of stairs before work to be more alert to start the work-day.

My mental goal is _____.

3. Physical performance goals refer to how activity can aid in developing more energy and physical skills.

Example: I will hike as a way to increase stamina.

My physical performance goal is _____.

4. Health goals refer to how activity can aid in reducing health risk.

Example: I will walk vigorously as a way to lose weight.

My health goal is _____.

From *Fit for Duty, Second Edition*, by Robert Hoffman and Thomas R. Collingwood, 2005, Champaign, IL: Human Kinetics.

Assessing your level of physical activity provides a quick picture of where you are. The act of defining goals helps crystallize exactly why you want to engage in physical activity and helps define where you want to be.

Neutralizing Barriers

The third step is to review potential barriers to being physically active. Barriers are those obstacles that can keep us from starting and following a physical activity program. It's not always easy to change habits or start a new behavior. It can seem that there is never a "good" time to change. In this day of the information age, we always seem to be too busy or too inundated with commitments and responsibilities. Yet most barriers can be overcome if being active can be made a personal priority.

Barriers to exercising can be physical, social, or psychological. Identifying those barriers and planning to minimize them before starting a program greatly enhances the probability for success. You defined some of those barriers when you weighed the advantages and disadvantages of starting a program. Some of the more common barriers and how they can be neutralized are as follows:

- **Inconvenience.** If doing an activity is not convenient, we are less apt to make the effort. To minimize this barrier, try to select a location for your activity that is easy to get to and safe. You will have more difficulty sustaining a program if you have to travel great distances or the location is not in a safe area. Activity locations near your home or workplace enhance adherence. Likewise, selecting a location in a safe area or choosing a time of day when safety is more assured is prudent.

- **Physical environment.** The weather may be too hot, too cold, or too wet. Timing of activity is one way to neutralize this factor. For example, you might choose to walk early in the morning before the heat and humidity become too uncomfortable. Or you could seek out a location such as a mall where the environment is controlled.

- **Lack of time.** Lack of time is probably the most popular excuse for not being active. Family, friends, and work obligations all compete for your time, and shift work can be a major problem. However, surveys indicate that some of the busiest people, including U.S. presidents and corporate executives, are able to find time for an exercise program. If they can find the time, most of us should be able to do so as well. It's a matter of making time for yourself and making physical activity a priority. There are 168 waking hours in a week. Using basic time management skills such as evaluating when you have idle time can aid in finding time to do physical activity. For example, taking an extra 30 minutes before or after a shift to go walking may be doable for many officers.

- **Injury.** A preexisting injury can be a barrier. For example, having a back problem may make yard work uncomfortable and painful. In such cases, selecting an activity that doesn't aggravate an injury becomes critical. For example, moderate walking or cycling can be performed even with back problems. Another way to minimize the injury factor is to be sure to warm up before performing an activity.

- **Lack of skill.** Activities such as racquetball or tennis require certain motor skills. If you lack a particular skill, you probably won't enjoy the activity and may even find it embarrassing to participate. Consequently, the activity will not be sustained. Lack of skill may be a barrier to participation for certain activities, but it need not keep you from participating in other activities requiring less skill, such as walking. Likewise, if you really want to learn an activity but lack the skills, you can look for opportunities to get instruction at local recreation centers.

- **Social or cultural.** Sometimes our circle of family, friends, and coworkers are not active and may not be very supportive of our efforts to change behavior. You may have to go it alone, which for many of us can be a barrier. One option is to try to find a physical activity club or class to join. Another way to overcome this barrier is to find a partner who is also willing to exercise.

You may identify other personal barriers that need to be explored. The key is recognizing that your activity level, your fitness, and your health are priorities. With that in mind—"where there is a will there is a way."

CREATING A PLAN

"Get ready. Get set. Go!" are the ageless instructions for starting a race. Initiating action is the "Go!" command. There are three steps in starting physical activity:

- Incorporating activity into daily living
- Structuring a physical activity plan
- Committing to a walking preassessment program

Incorporating Activity Into Daily Living

This step involves nothing more than looking for opportunities to expend energy in physical activity. Some simple examples are taking the stairs instead of an elevator; moving around the house or office whenever possible; instead of calling to people in other rooms, getting up to go see them; and throwing away the TV remote. Rather than employing someone to do the yard work all the time, do it yourself occasionally. Some people deliberately park their car several blocks from work so that they have to walk to and from the office. If you think through a typical day, you will find ample opportunities to expend more energy.

Another approach to being more active is to decrease sedentary activities. A simple guideline is to stand instead of sitting and walk instead of standing. Although there is nothing wrong with sedentary activities such as reading and watching TV, there are substitute activities. For example, you could get audio books and listen to a book while walking. Instead of sitting around and talking when visiting friends, try doing a "walk and talk" together. The bottom line is that by seeking opportunities to be more active and expend energy, a movement habit will develop that will help set the stage for more formal and structured activity.

Structuring a Physical Activity Plan

Seeking opportunities to be more active and trying to be less sedentary are informal ways of being more physically active. However, by designing a physical activity plan and writing it down, you make it more likely that physical activity will become a sustained behavior or habit for you.

The ACSM has recommended that engaging in some form of light or moderate physical activity for at least 30 minutes on most days of the week is the minimum amount (or threshold) for seeing improved physical function and health benefits. This is the equivalent of burning approximately 1,000 calories a week through physical exercise. The activity should be strenuous enough to rev up your breathing and heart rate. There are four steps to defining the plan.

1. Select an activity or activities based on what you like to do, what is convenient, and what can be readily substituted for sedentary behaviors at home, work, or school.

2. List the days of the week on which you will do each activity.
3. List the duration of and times when you will do the activity.
4. List where you will do the activity.

A sample activity plan is shown below.

Sample Activity Plan

Activity	What days	When	Where
Walk part of beat area	Monday-Friday	Randomly for 15 minutes	Five blocks around beat area
Gardening	Saturday	1:00 to 1:30	Home
Walk	Monday-Sunday	After dinner for 15 minutes	Eight blocks around home
Use stairs, not elevator	Monday-Friday	During workday	At the station

You can see from the example that the 30-minutes-a-day goal can be achieved through different activities and does not have to be done all at once. Use the blank form below to create your own activity plan.

My Activity Plan

Activity	What days	When	Where
_____	_____	_____	_____
_____	_____	_____	_____
_____	_____	_____	_____
_____	_____	_____	_____
_____	_____	_____	_____

From *Fit for Duty, Second Edition*, by Robert Hoffman and Thomas R. Collingwood, 2005, Champaign, IL: Human Kinetics.

Walking Preassessment Starter Program

If you answered yes to any of the Par-Q questions or if you had some additional screening that suggests you may have some activity risk, we recommend that you perform an eight-week starter walking program before taking the fitness assessments. The following walking program is a gradually progressive program. Do the following each time you walk:

- Warm up before you start your walk by swinging your arms and performing mild stretches. Chapters 5 and 7 will provide more information on warm-up activities.
- Start slowly, then pick up the pace. Walk briskly without getting out of breath.
- Slow your pace for the last 2 minutes to serve as a cool-down.

The most important variable is the duration (time). Use the distance as a goal for each week. The chart below shows how long you should walk each week.

Eight-Week Walking Program

Week	Goal distance	Goal duration (minutes)	Frequency per week
1	1/2 mile	12:00	3-4
2	3/4 mile	18:00	3-4
3	1 mile	23:00	3-4
4	1 mile	23:00	3-4
5	1.25 mile	23:00	4
6	1.5 miles	26:00	4
7	1.5 miles	26:00	4-5
8	2.0 miles	33:00	4-5

If you find that the plan for week 1 is too easy, start the program at a level you are comfortable with. Once you have completed week 8, test yourself with the 1-mile walk test (outlined on the following page). The results will help you determine if you are ready for the regular fitness assessments.

FOLLOWING THE PLAN

The final step is to follow your program. Here are a few tips that may help.

- Keep a log of how often you do the various activities. This can help keep your program on track.
- Look for a way to reward yourself after following the program for a set time period, such as a month.
- Seek out sources that will support your efforts. Try to find a friend, family member, or coworker to do some of the activities with you and help you with your efforts. Since walking is a popular and easy activity, you could conduct

One-Mile Walk

The one-mile walk test will determine how well your walking program has prepared you for the more strenuous fitness tests. In this test, you measure the time it takes to walk a mile and your heart rate at the end of the test.

Equipment

- Stopwatch
- 440-yard track or marked level course

Procedure

1. Walk 1 mile as fast as possible. Running or jogging are not permitted.
2. When you finish the mile, note your time and immediately find either your radial or carotid pulse. Take your pulse for 6 seconds and multiply the count by 10. (You must measure your pulse as soon as you cross the finish line to get an accurate exercise heart rate.)
3. Cool down by walking slowly for 5 minutes.
4. Compare your time and heart rate with the norms in table 2.1. Find the column for your age and gender category and match up your posttest pulse rate with the closest standard rate on the left side of the chart. You may need to make an adjustment if your weight differs from the specified weight.
5. Note that there are age differences for a given heart rate. The reason for this disparity is that maximum heart rate decreases with age, which means that a younger person is working at a lower level of cardiovascular endurance than an older individual would be at the same heart rate.
6. If your time for the 1-mile walk is equal to or less than the time corresponding to your heart rate, you can feel confident that you can safely take the fitness tests in chapter 3. If not, you should stay with week 8 of the program for an additional four weeks and retest.

TABLE 2.1 One-Mile Walk Norms

Heart rate	MEN (Assumes a weight of 175 pounds*)					WOMEN (Assumes a weight of 125 pounds*)				
	20-29	30-39	40-49	50-59	60+	20-29	30-39	40-49	50-59	60+
110	19:36	18:21	18:05	17:49	17:55	20:57	19:46	19:15	18:40	18:00
120	19:10	17:52	17:36	17:20	17:24	20:27	19:18	18:45	18:12	17:30
130	18:35	17:22	17:07	16:51	16:57	20:00	18:48	18:18	17:42	17:01
140	18:06	16:54	16:38	16:22	16:28	19:30	18:18	17:48	17:18	16:31
150	17:36	16:26	16:09	15:53	15:59	19:00	17:48	17:18	16:48	16:02
160	17:19	15:58	15:42	15:26	15:30	18:30	17:18	16:48	16:18	15:32
170	16:39	15:28	15:12	14:56	15:04	18:00	16:54	16:18	15:48	15:04

* For every 10 pounds over 175 pounds, men must walk 15 seconds faster to meet the standard; for every 10 pounds under 175 pounds, men can walk 15 seconds slower to meet the standard.

* For every 10 pounds over 125 pounds, women must walk 15 seconds faster to meet the standard; for every 10 pounds under 125 pounds, women can walk 15 seconds slower to meet the standard.

Adapted from Cooper Institute for Aerobic Research, 1990, *The strength connection* (Dallas, TX: Cooper Institute for Aerobic Research), 117-120.

"walking meetings" with coworkers, organize a neighborhood walking group, or set aside time to walk and talk with your spouse.

- Purchase a pedometer to measure the distance you walk. Using one can provide immediate feedback for tracking your walking distance.

Developing a new behavior requires getting ready, making a commitment, and getting started. Following this process enables you to become more physically active. Once this lifestyle choice becomes a habit, you can consider a more structured and strenuous exercise program that will further maximize the health benefits and significantly improve your physical fitness level. Now set a date for starting your physical activity program and keep it.

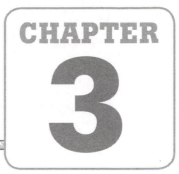
How Fit Are You?

After reading chapter 2, you may have recognized that you need a fitness program. Or if you're feeling that your fitness level is satisfactory, you may have skipped ahead to this chapter. Or you may just be unsure where you stand. In any case, the assessment instruments described in this chapter will help you determine your fitness status more precisely.

Some of you will be using this book to develop your own fitness program, and others will be using it under the guidance of a fitness coordinator or instructor. If you are in the latter group, this chapter may not apply to you right now, but you might want to familiarize yourself with its content in case you need to develop a program someday, either for yourself or for someone else. It may also help you to better understand your agency's assessment process.

IMPORTANCE OF TESTING

When some officers hear the words *fitness program,* the first thing they think of is a fitness test. Fitness tests alone do not get people fit enough to perform their jobs, but they do have an important place in the program.

Your agency may have validated a fitness test and standard. The purpose of the test in your case is to give you, your agency, and the public reasonable assurance that you are fit enough to cope with the physical requirements of the job at a minimum level of safety and effectiveness. Periodic testing provides a safe, controlled environment in which to identify those officers who may need additional training.

Most agencies do not have minimum fitness requirements for their incumbents. Assessing your level of fitness may be an individual responsibility. You may choose to measure your levels of fitness simply to compare your performance with that of other law enforcement officers. Or you may choose to use the results of the assessments to gauge the success of your training. In that case, you are likely to repeat the assessments at intervals to see if you are improving.

In any case, how many push-ups you can do for the sake of doing push-ups or how fast you can do a 1.5-mile run for the sake of running fast is not important. We know that the job requires some level of muscular strength and endurance, flexibility, cardiovascular endurance, and anaerobic power. The assessments give you relatively simple ways to measure your current level of fitness in each of these areas.

AGENCY FITNESS TESTING

Depending on your agency's program, you may be tested periodically for fitness. If so, you already have an idea of your fitness status. Once you know your score for each event, you can refer to chapter 14 for guidance on setting goals appropriate to your level of fitness.

The law enforcement agencies that administer physical fitness tests use either a fitness battery or a job task simulation test. Fitness batteries measure the components of physical fitness discussed in chapter 1. A typical fitness battery consists of tests such as the 1.5-mile run (cardiovascular endurance), one-repetition maximum (1RM) bench press (muscular strength), sit-ups and push-ups (muscular endurance), sit-and-reach test (flexibility), 300-meter run (anaerobic power), Illinois agility run (agility), vertical jump (explosive leg power), and skinfold measurements (body fat). These components of fitness underlie all physical tasks performed by law enforcement officers.

Law Enforcement Physical Standards

The first physical requirements in law enforcement were height and weight standards. Agencies were unable to defend these standards as job related and consistent with business necessity when challenged by certain groups, most notably women. Thus, they began developing obstacle-type courses that we call job task simulation tests. Although these tests looked like tasks officers did on the job, the standards were usually made up, and agencies could not defend them. About this time, The Cooper Institute (CI) took the lead in training fitness leaders for law enforcement. Officers attending the training were exposed to the large database the CI had developed. This database was displayed in 10-year groupings for both men and women. Because the fitness tests used by the CI were valid measures of the components of fitness, some agencies began using this test battery. However, the fitness test norms were based on a select population that did not include any law enforcement officers. Likewise, the norms are not a true representation of the fitness levels of the general population. Unfortunately, many of the agencies using those fitness tests also adopted the age- and gender-based normative data as standards. Since the job requirements are not based on age or gender, it doesn't make sense to have different fitness standards for different groups of people doing the same job. Furthermore, Title VII of the Civil Rights Acts prohibits using different cutoff scores for employment decisions based on race, color, religion, national origin, or gender. So whichever type of test your agency selects, the test and standard must be defensible as being job related, and the standard must be the same for everyone taking the test.

Job task simulation tests, sometimes called ability or agility tests, consist of a series of physical tasks that law enforcement officers would typically perform. You might think of such a test as an obstacle course. For example, a test may be run over a 300-meter course that includes climbing a fence, jumping over a ditch, crawling through a culvert, and dragging a weighted dummy. One drawback of job task simulation tests is that they typically account for only 20 to 25 percent of the physical tasks performed by law enforcement officers.

Either type of test is acceptable from a job-related validity perspective. The experience of many professionals in the field, including the staffs of the CI and FitForce, is that fitness testing is a much better measure of the underlying factors predicting who can and cannot perform the essential physical tasks of law enforcement work.

Regardless of which type of test your agency uses, the more important factor is having a fitness program. The test can give you a starting point for your program and evaluate its effectiveness, but the program itself is what makes you perform your job better.

ASSESSING YOUR FITNESS LEVEL

If your agency does not currently administer a fitness test, the following fitness assessment is relatively simple to administer and score and will give you enough information about your fitness level to start a program. To complete the assessment, you will need a stopwatch, a box, a yardstick, a piece of chalk, four traffic cones, a mat, a bench press machine or free weights and a bench (if you only have free weights, you will need to enlist a couple of friends to serve as spotters), and a track or other area to walk or run a known distance. You may also want a helper to run the stopwatch and record scores. Your local high school probably has a track, and that would be a good place to do the test. Record your results on the Physical Fitness Assessment Sheet on page 38. You might want to make copies of this form to record your progress on retests.

You will learn how to perform the fitness tests in the pages that follow. Our research shows that all components of fitness are important for the performance of law enforcement work; however, you may be unable to complete all of the assessments due to lack of facilities, or you may choose to select only certain measures. In either case, enter the raw score for each event you complete in the space provided on the Physical Fitness Assessment Sheet. Refer to table 3.1 on page 39 to see how you compare with other law enforcement officers. You may choose to record the fitness percentile categories in the space provided.

Before taking any of the fitness tests, you should review your Par-Q from chapter 2. If you answered yes to any questions, have you cleared those issues with your doctor or fitness coordinator? Second, review how well your starter program has been progressing. Have you been able to stick with the starter plan? Has the physical activity been too easy or too hard? If you have followed the starter program and the activity was not too difficult, you are ready for the fitness tests. If you have not taken the 1-mile walk test described in chapter 2, you need to do so before taking the fitness assessments. If your time for the 1-mile walk was equal to or less than the time on the chart for your heart rate, it should be safe for you to take the fitness tests. If not, we recommend that you stay with the week 8 program for an additional four weeks and retest.

Physical Fitness Assessment Sheet

Screening tests	Screening test scores
1. Height	_____ inches
2. Weight	_____ pounds
3. Resting heart rate	_____ beats per minute
4. Resting blood pressure	_____ mm/Hg
5. Cholesterol (if available)	_____ mg/dl

Fitness tests	Fitness test scores	Fitness level
1. 1.5-mile run	_____ min:sec	_____
2. 300-meter run	_____ seconds	_____
3. 1RM bench press	_____ pounds	_____
	_____ ratio (weight pressed divided by body weight)	
4. 1-minute sit-up	_____ (number completed)	_____
5. Maximum push-up	_____ (number completed)	_____
6. Vertical jump	_____ inches	_____
7. Illinois agility run	_____ seconds	_____
8. Sit-and-reach test	_____ inches	_____
9. Body mass index or percent fat	_____ BMI	_____
	_____ percent fat	_____

From *Fit for Duty, Second Edition*, by Robert Hoffman and Thomas R. Collingwood, 2005, Champaign, IL: Human Kinetics.

In addition, you should avoid eating or smoking for at least an hour before beginning the test battery. If possible, get someone to help you with the test. You can administer it to yourself, but it will be easier if you have help.

Always warm up before physical activity. As a minimum, jog easily until you break a sweat. Then do about 5 minutes of stretching exercises, concentrating on the body parts to be exercised. See chapter 5 for more information about warm-up.

Give yourself at least two days to take all the tests. If possible, avoid doing the 1RM bench press and the maximum push-up test on the same day. Likewise, consider doing the 1.5-mile run and the 300-meter run on different days. If you are using the results of your assessment to evaluate the progress of your training program, the primary consideration is to conduct the reassessments using the same schedule. Here is a sample test schedule.

Day 1

1RM bench press
1-minute sit-up test
Illinois agility run
Sit-and-reach test
300-meter run

Day 2

Vertical jump
Maximum push-up test
1.5-mile run

TABLE 3.1 FitForce Law Enforcement Physical Fitness Norms

Percentile	1.5-mile run	300-meter run	1RM bench press (raw)	1RM bench press (ratio)	Push-up	Sit-up	Vertical jump	Agility	Sit-and-reach	% fat	% FAT Men	% FAT Women
High												
99th	9:28	38.8	355	1.75	77	60	28	15.2	26	6.2	5.7	8.9
90th	11:31	48.3	273	1.38	56	49	23	16.2	23	12.7	11.8	17.5
80th	12:32	52.8	243	1.23	47	44	21	16.7	21	15.7	14.3	20.3
70th	13:14	55.6	220	1.12	40	40	20	17.0	20	17.3	16.4	22.2
Moderate												
60th	13:58	58.9	202	1.02	35	37	19	17.3	19	19.0	18.1	23.9
50th	14:40	62.2	182	0.93	31	34	18	17.7	18	20.5	19.6	25.4
40th	15:20	65.4	163	0.86	29	31	16	18.0	17	22.0	21.1	27.0
30th	15:55	70.1	153	0.79	24	28	15	18.5	16	23.7	22.9	24.0
Low												
20th	16:55	75.3	133	0.71	19	25	14	19.1	15	25.3	25.0	31.1
10th	17:00	82.9	104	0.60	13	20	12	20.1	13	28.3	28.1	34.4
1st	23:35	114.7	60	0.40	2	6	7	24.3	9	34.8	36.8	44.2

Qualitative scores can be applied to BMI scores with the ranges for health-related BMI below:

Health index	BMI score (men and women)
Underweight	18.5
Ideal	18.5 to 24.9
Overweight	25.0 to 29.9
Obese	30.0 to 39.9
Extremely obese	40 and above

One-Repetition Maximum (1RM) Bench Press

This test measures the amount of force the upper body can generate. The score is the maximum weight pushed from the bench press position. The 1RM is important for measuring your ability to perform tasks requiring upper body strength, such as pushing, lifting, and carrying, and in use-of-force situations.

There are two options for testing 1RM. Actual maximum testing requires you to lift as much weight as possible in one repetition. You can also estimate your maximum using a submaximal effort. If you have not lifted weights within the past year, we recommend doing the submaximal testing to lessen your chances of injury.

Equipment

- A free weight set or chest press machine. For consistency, only one or the other should be used. If a chest press machine is used and there are two sets of numbers for a given plate, use the higher number.

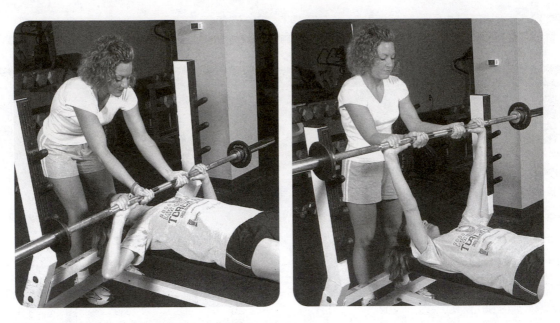

Proper bench press positions: start and lifted.

Procedures if maximum testing is performed

1. Use a spotter if free weights are used.
2. Estimate the weight that you can press in one maximum effort. Start with about two-thirds of that weight. If you are unable to estimate your maximum, start with 50 percent of your body weight if you are male and 25 percent of your body weight if you are female.
3. Have the spotters lift the weight from the stand and hold it until you are in control of the bar. Press this weight several times for an easy warm-up.
4. Increase the weight in 10-pound or greater increments to maximum. Five-pound increments may be more appropriate as you get closer to maximum. Lift each additional weight increment starting from the down position. The first three to four repetitions serve as warm-up lifts to prevent muscle injury and to prepare you for a maximal lift on the *fifth* or *sixth* effort.
5. The score for this test is the maximum number of pounds lifted in one repetition.
6. Divide the 1RM score by your body weight to get your 1RM ratio score.
7. Record the score on your Physical Fitness Assessment Sheet.
8. If using a bench press machine, spotters may not be necessary. Most bench press machines are designed so that you must start in the down position. Note that the bench press norms in table 3.1 were developed using free weights, making comparisons to weights lifted using machines irrelevant.

Procedures if estimated weights are used

1. Set the weight at 60 percent of body weight for men and 30 percent for women.
2. Do as many repetitions as possible.
3. Use table 3.2 to determine your estimated 1RM maximum by locating the intersection between the weight used and the number of repetitions you performed.

TABLE 3.2　Estimated 1RM Weights

1RM	2 reps	4 reps	6 reps	8 reps	10 reps	12 reps	14 reps	16 reps	18 reps	20 reps
200	190	180	170	160	150	140	130	120	110	100
195	185	175	165	156	146	136	126	117	107	97
190	180	171	161	152	142	133	123	114	104	95
185	175	166	157	148	138	129	120	111	101	92
180	171	162	153	144	135	126	117	108	99	90
175	166	157	148	140	131	122	113	105	96	87
170	161	153	144	136	127	119	110	102	93	86
165	156	148	140	132	123	115	107	99	90	82
160	152	144	136	128	120	112	104	96	88	80
155	147	139	131	124	116	108	100	93	85	77
150	142	135	127	120	112	105	97	90	82	75
145	137	130	123	116	108	101	94	87	79	72
140	133	126	119	112	105	98	91	84	77	70
135	128	121	114	108	101	94	87	81	74	67
130	123	117	110	104	97	91	84	78	71	65
125	118	112	106	100	93	87	81	75	68	62
120	114	108	102	96	90	84	78	72	66	60
115	109	103	97	92	86	80	74	69	63	57
110	104	99	93	88	82	77	71	66	60	55
105	99	94	89	84	78	73	68	63	57	52
100	95	90	85	80	75	70	65	60	55	50
95	90	85	80	76	71	66	61	57	52	47
90	85	81	76	72	67	63	58	54	49	45
85	80	76	72	68	63	59	55	51	46	42
80	76	72	68	64	60	56	52	48	44	40
75	71	67	63	60	56	52	48	45	41	37
70	66	63	59	56	52	49	45	42	38	35
65	61	58	55	52	48	45	42	39	35	32
60	57	54	51	48	45	42	39	36	33	30
55	52	49	46	44	41	38	35	33	30	27
50	47	45	42	40	37	35	32	30	27	25
45	42	40	38	36	33	31	29	27	24	22
40	38	36	34	32	30	28	26	24	22	20
35	33	31	29	28	26	24	22	21	19	17
30	28	27	25	24	22	21	19	18	16	15
25	23	22	21	20	19	17	16	15	14	12
20	19	18	17	16	15	14	13	12	11	10
15	10	9	8	8	7	7	6	6	5	5
10	5	5	4	4	4	4	3	3	3	2

Adapted from P.O. Davis, 1996, *Fitness coordinator's manual,* 12th ed. (Burtonville, MD: ARA/Hillman Factors, Inc.)

4. If you were able to do more than 20 repetitions of a given weight, take a 5-minute rest period, add 10 to 15 pounds, and do as many repetitions as possible with the new weight.

5. Determine your ratio score by dividing the estimated weight pressed by your body weight.

One-Minute Sit-Up Test

This test measures abdominal muscle endurance, which is important for performing tasks that involve use of force and helps maintain good posture and minimize lower back problems. The score is the number of sit-ups completed in 1 minute. This test should be performed on grass, a mat, or a carpeted surface.

Equipment

- A mat, if desired
- A stopwatch
- A helper

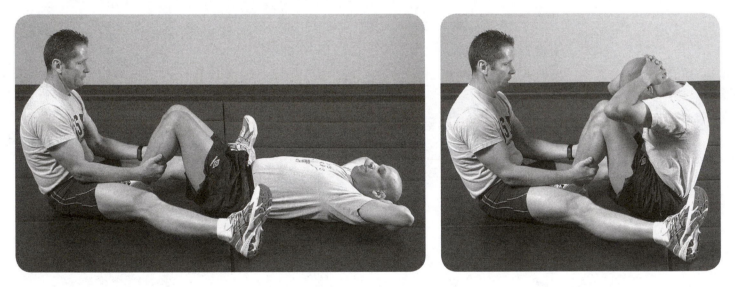

Proper sit-up positions: start and up.

Procedures

1. Lie on your back with your knees bent and your heels flat on the mat or ground. Your hands should be held to the sides of your head, the fingertips behind your ears, with your elbows out to the sides. Your partner should hold down your feet. If a helper is not available, put your feet under a couch or similar item to anchor them.

2. Bending at the waist, sit up until your elbows touch or pass your knees, and then return to a full lying position before starting the next sit-up. You may rest in either the starting or up position.

3. Do as many correct sit-ups as possible in 1 minute.

4. The score for this test is the number of correct sit-ups performed. Record your score on the Physical Fitness Assessment Sheet.

The Sit-Up Controversy

Over the years, we have found the sit-up to be the most controversial of the fitness tests. A commonly held perception is that interlocking the fingers behind the head will strain the neck, perhaps causing injury. We have administered thousands of sit-up tests and have never seen this happen; however, to preclude these concerns, we have changed the test protocol to allow that only the tips of the fingers remain behind the ears.

A little-known fact is that the abdominals only work as far as your spine can bend. The hip flexors and iliopsoas do the rest of the work in moving the torso to the sitting position. Therefore, when *training* to develop abdominal endurance, crunches are a better choice. But testing abdominal endurance using crunches has drawbacks. Not everyone's spine flexes to the same degree, making it difficult to know if an individual has come to their maximum "up" position. For this reason, during *testing,* we have continued to require that the elbows touch or pass the knees. Also, to standardize testing, we require that the feet be anchored; for training, we recommend that they not be anchored.

Agility Run

This test is a measure of coordinated movement and speed, an important area for performing tasks requiring quick movements around obstacles. The score is the time it takes to complete a 180-foot serpentine course.

Equipment

- Four cones
- A marked course (cones placed 10 feet apart in a straight line for a total distance of 30 feet)
- A stopwatch

Procedures

1. Lie prone on the ground with your hands on the starting line to the left of the line of cones.
2. To start, stand up and sprint to the last cone (30 feet away), place one foot over the line, then sprint back to the starting line.
3. Make a left turn around the first cone, then zigzag in a figure-eight fashion around the four cones and back to the starting line.
4. Then sprint up and back as described in step 2.
5. The score for this test is your time to the nearest tenth of a second.
6. Take two trials. Use the best score (lowest time) of the two.
7. Record your score on the Physical Fitness Assessment Sheet.

Sit-and-Reach Test

This test measures the flexibility of the lower back and upper leg area, which is important for performing tasks involving range of motion and in minimizing lower back problems. The score is recorded to the nearest half inch.

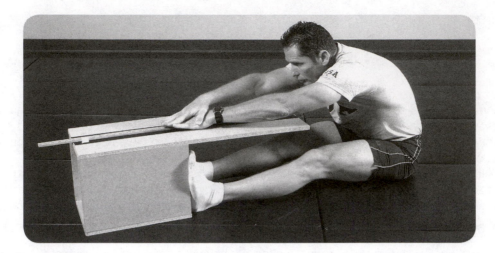

Proper sit-and-reach position.

Equipment

- A 12-inch-high box
- A yardstick attached to the top of the box, with the 15-inch mark at the edge of the box and the 36-inch mark pointing away from you
- A helper (mandatory)

Procedures

1. Warm up slowly by practicing the test.
2. Sit on the ground or mat with your shoes off and your legs extended at right angles to the box. Keep your legs straight. Your heels should touch the near edge of the box and should be 8 inches apart. The yardstick should be centered over the space between your legs.
3. Slowly reach forward with both hands (one on top of the other) as far as possible and hold the position momentarily. Have your helper note the distance your fingertips reach on the yardstick to the nearest half inch.
4. The best of three trials is your score. Record your score on the Physical Fitness Assessment Sheet.

300-Meter Run

This is a test of anaerobic capacity, which is important for short, intense bursts of effort such as in pursuit tasks. The score is the time it takes to complete a 300-meter course.

Equipment

- A marked course of 300 meters (328 yards, or 984 feet)
- A stopwatch

Procedures

1. Warm up by jogging slowly for 2 minutes and stretching.
2. At the "Go" signal, run as fast as possible for the course duration.
3. Record your time on the Physical Fitness Assessment Sheet.

Vertical Jump

This test is a measure of jumping or explosive power, an important area for pursuit tasks that require jumping and vaulting. The score is the difference in inches between your standing and jumping reach heights.

Equipment

- A yardstick taped to a smooth wall
- Chalk dust or chalk for marking standing and jumping reach heights

Procedures

1. Stand with one side toward the wall and reach up as high as possible to mark your standing reach height.
2. Take one step back and jump as high as possible, and mark the spot on the wall above your standing reach mark. You may also jump with both feet.
3. Your score is the difference in inches (to the nearest 1/2 inch) between your standing and jumping reach heights.
4. Use the best score of three trials.
5. Record your score on the Physical Fitness Assessment Sheet.

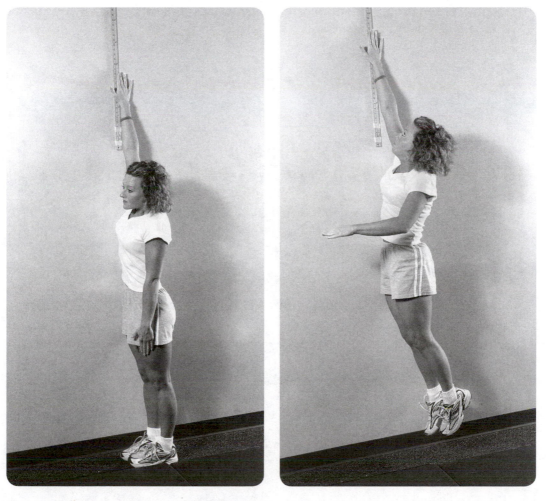

Proper vertical jump positions: starting and jumping.

Maximum Push-Up Test

This test measures the muscular endurance of the upper body muscles used in pushing, lifting, carrying, and use-of-force situations. Your score is the maximum number of push-ups you can perform.

Equipment

- A helper, if available

Procedures

1. Get down on the floor into the front-leaning rest position. Place your palms on the ground, approximately shoulder-width apart, with your back straight and your feet approximately 8 inches apart.

2. Your helper (if you have one) should crouch in front of you and ensure that your upper arms are parallel to the ground each time you lower yourself before returning to the starting position.

3. Lower your body by bending your elbows until your upper arms are parallel with the ground; then push up again. Keep your back straight, and in each upward extension, lock your elbows.

4. Rest in the up position.

5. The score is the number of correct push-ups completed. Record your score on the Physical Fitness Assessment Sheet.

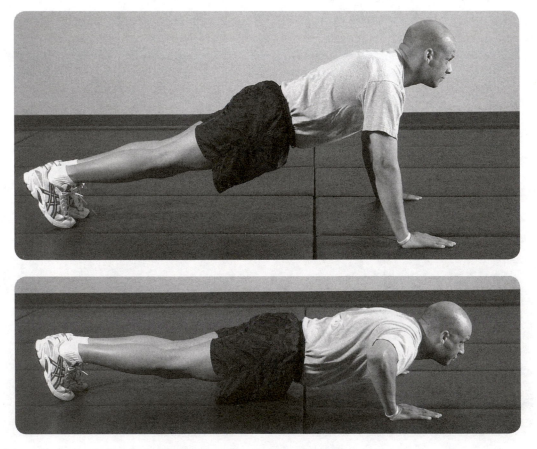

Proper push-up positions: start and lowered.

1.5-Mile Run

This run is a measure of cardiovascular endurance or aerobic power, which is important in foot pursuits and use-of-force encounters lasting more than 2 minutes. The score is the time it takes to complete the 1.5-mile course.

Equipment

- A track or marked level course
- A stopwatch
- A helper, if available

Procedures

Before testing, measure out a course of exactly 1.5 miles. A quarter-mile running track is ideal. *Note:* Make sure you know if the track is 440 yards or 400 meters. If using a 400-meter track, you must run six laps plus 14 meters, or 15 yards, to equal 1.5 miles.

1. Warm up and stretch before the run.
2. Have your helper give the "Go" signal and begin timing you. If you don't have a helper, start the watch yourself as you begin running.
3. Run the distance as fast as possible. Note your time at the end of the run.
4. Cool down by walking for an additional 5 minutes or so. Cooling down helps speed up the return of blood to the heart, reducing the chances of fainting. (See more on warm-up and cool-down in chapter 5.)
5. The score is the time it takes to run the course. Record your score on the Physical Fitness Assessment Sheet.

Body Composition

This assessment estimates your fat-to-lean ratio or your height-to-weight ratio. A good fat-to-lean ratio is important to both health and performance. Leaner people tend to perform physical tasks better and with less fatigue. Maintaining lower levels of body fat lessens your chances of developing diseases such as heart problems, diabetes, and certain cancers.

Procedures

Body composition can be estimated in several ways. A professional can perform the assessment using underwater weighing, skinfold measurements using calipers, or electrical impedance measurements. You can calculate your body mass index by yourself. If you are able to get an assessment of body fat, record the amount on the Physical Fitness Assessment Sheet.

Calculating BMI

1. Determine your weight in pounds and your height in inches.
2. Square your height in inches.
3. Divide your weight by your height (in inches) squared.
4. Multiply the result of step 3 by 703 to get your BMI.
5. Record your BMI on the Physical Fitness Assessment Sheet.

USING YOUR TEST RESULTS

Once you have completed the tests, you may want to compare the results with the FitForce norms in table 3.1. These norms are based on tests of more than 4,000 law enforcement officers throughout the United States. The norms are arranged by percentile. The 50th percentile is approximately the same as the average score. If your score for a particular test was at the 30th percentile, it means that 70 percent of the officers in the sample performed better than you did. Similarly, it means that you performed better than 30 percent of the officers in the sample. Find your score in the appropriate table, determine the fitness level for your percentile (high, moderate, low) for each event, and write it in the designated space on the Physical Fitness Assessment Sheet. Sample results for an officer with moderate and low levels of fitness are shown below. As noted earlier, since the tasks police officers must perform are the same regardless of age or gender, the same norms should be used for all law enforcement officers.

In subsequent chapters, you'll learn how to use the results of your assessment to establish goals and develop a fitness program. Now that you have a feel for your current level of fitness, you'll learn more about each component of physical fitness and how to develop a program to help improve your performance in your weak areas.

Sample Fitness Results

Screening tests	Scores	
1. Height	72 inches	
2. Weight	230 pounds	
3. Resting heart rate	80 beats per minute	
4. Resting blood pressure	140/88 mm/Hg	
5. Cholesterol (if available)	250 mg/dl	

Fitness tests	Fitness test score	Fitness level
1. 1.5-mile run	16:00 min:sec	Low
2. 300-meter run	75 seconds	Low
3. 1RM bench press	210 pounds	Moderate
	0.91 ratio (weight pressed divided by body weight	Moderate
4. 1-minute sit-up test	26 completed	Low
5. Maximum push-up test	20 completed	Low
6. Vertical jump	14 inches	Low
7. Illinois agility run	18.5 seconds	Moderate
8. Sit-and-reach test	17 inches	Moderate
9. Body mass index or percent fat	31.2 BMI	Obese
	25 percent fat	Low

Training for Fitness

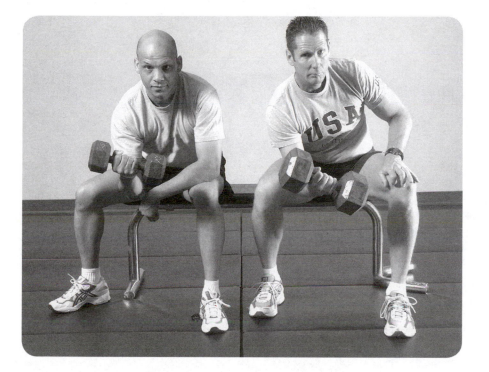

In part I, you learned what the components of physical fitness are and assessed your own level of fitness. In part II, you will learn more about the importance of the physical fitness components and how to train in each of the areas. When you finish this part of the book, you will have the knowledge you need to design an exercise program that will improve your cardiovascular endurance, anaerobic power, muscular strength and endurance, and flexibility. These activities, along with what you will learn later about diet and nutrition, will enable you to change your body composition, lowering the amount of fat and adding lean muscle mass. These improvements will take time and will require you to make changes in your behaviors, but they will enhance your performance and health.

In chapter 4, we discuss the principles of exercise. The information about the principles of exercise applies equally well to the beginner and to more experienced exercisers. In chapters 5 through 8, we discuss the components of physical fitness and tell you how to train for each and what activities to use. You will learn the acronym FITT, which will help you remember how to apply the principles of exercise to each component of physical fitness.

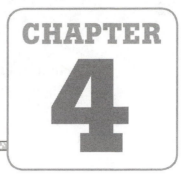

Principles of Exercise

As with other sciences, the science of exercise has principles that have been developed through observation and research and substantiated through practice. The principles of exercise tell you how to exercise correctly and safely. You may see different combinations or lists in other fitness books, but the principles you'll learn here are selected for their appropriateness to law enforcement officers, although they could apply to any group of exercisers. When designing your fitness program, the following 11 principles of exercise should be considered:

Regularity	Variety
Recovery	Specificity
Reversibility	Adaptation
Overload	Individuality
Progression	Moderation
Balance	

In addition to considering all 11 principles of exercise, you need to know how often, how hard, and how long to exercise and what activities will produce a training effect. To help you remember this information, we use the acronym FITT.

Frequency—How often to perform the type of exercise. Frequency incorporates the principles of regularity, recovery, and reversibility.

Intensity—How hard to exercise. Intensity incorporates the principles of overload and progression.

Time—How long an exercise session should be. Time also incorporates the principles of overload and progression.

Type—What types of activities train each component. Type incorporates the principles of balance, variety, and specificity.

In the next few chapters, we will apply the principles of exercise to each of the components of physical fitness. You will learn the FITT for each fitness component and will see more specifically how the principles relate to your training plan. You don't need to memorize the list of principles. Instead, the important thing is to understand the concepts they represent. That knowledge will ensure that your fitness program is safe and effective.

PRINCIPLE 1: REGULARITY

The weekend-warrior approach to fitness training will probably produce more injuries than desirable results. To be effective, a fitness program must be followed regularly. Trying to get all the training you need in irregular bursts doesn't work. Rather, your training should be consistent throughout the week, month, year, and your life.

Fitness research indicates that it takes a minimum of three exercise sessions per week to achieve cardiovascular training. Indications are that as few as two strength training sessions per week are necessary to see gains in that area. As you will see later, you should do at least some flexibility training each time you do any exercise.

Compare fitness training to marksmanship training. If the only time you fire your weapon is during requalification, your scores likely will go down. But if you have the opportunity to practice between qualifications, you are likely to improve. Although it is important to train at least the minimum number of times for each of the fitness components each training week, you don't want to overtrain.

Experts tell us that an energy system or muscle group will begin to decondition after 96 hours of inactivity. Although this change will be imperceptible, it does give us a parameter for regularity. As a rule of thumb, plan your workouts so there is a maximum of 96 hours between hard training sessions for the same energy system or muscle group.

PRINCIPLE 2: RECOVERY

The body needs time to recover between strenuous exercise sessions. As a general rule, allow 48 hours for recovery between hard workouts. For example, if you lift weights for the upper body on Monday, you should wait until Wednesday before training those muscles again. However, working out the lower body on Tuesday will not violate this principle.

Along with recovering between exercise sessions, you need to get sufficient sleep and allow for recovery from peak physical events such as your agency's fitness test or a race that you trained for. For most active people, getting 7 or 8 hours of sleep a night ensures sufficient rest for their lifestyle. When developing your

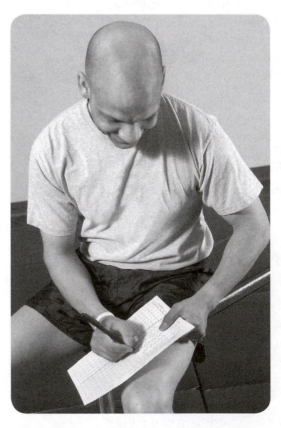

The frequency of physical activity is important.

long-range training plan, take into consideration that after an all-out effort for which you have trained extra hard, you should go a little easier for a while.

The threshold values for frequency of training (for example, three times a week for cardiovascular endurance [CVE]) were developed using a convention familiar to everyone. However, defining a week as a seven-day period beginning on Sunday and ending on Saturday does not always work for law enforcement officers. Your training week may be seven, eight, or even nine days long. The key is to make sure your training is regular and provides enough recovery time.

PRINCIPLE 3: REVERSIBILITY

Fitness is a "use it or lose it" proposition, and most training adaptations are reversible. It takes longer to achieve a level of fitness than it does to lose it. Some setbacks in your training regimen are unavoidable. Thus, the more "money in the bank" you have stored up, the more able you will be to withstand those periods when you are unable to train. You must maintain your training.

These principles of regularity, recovery, and reversibility relate to the F in FITT, which stands for the *frequency* of exercise necessary to achieve a training effect.

PRINCIPLE 4: OVERLOAD

For a training program to have an effect, the demands placed on the body must be greater than those of your day-to-day activities. You'll never improve your cardiovascular endurance if your most strenuous exercise is walking from the patrol car to the station house (although a brisk walk might produce a training effect). Nor will you increase your strength if you never overcome any more resistance than lifting a coffee cup. For each part of your program, as your fitness level improves, you must increase the demands of your training to ensure overload.

PRINCIPLE 5: PROGRESSION

There are two aspects to progression. One, as noted, is that as your level of fitness improves, you must increase the overload. The other is that these changes should be gradual. The story of the ancient Greek wrestler Milo illustrates both of these aspects. Milo trained in part by lifting a calf every day. As the calf grew into a cow, Milo's strength increased.

To improve your cardiovascular endurance, you must systematically train faster or longer, or both. To improve your strength, you must increase the resistance your muscles must overcome. As your body adapts to the current overload, you must progressively increase that overload to continue to improve.

The principles of overload and progression help us determine the *intensity* of exercise necessary to achieve a training effect, as well as how long each training session should last—the *time*.

One of the most important lessons we learned as fitness trainers is to progress *gradually*. There is a fine line between appropriate enthusiasm and trying to do too much too soon. The latter often results in soreness or injury and a greater likelihood of dropping out. When in doubt, increase the overload slower rather than faster.

PRINCIPLE 6: BALANCE

To achieve total fitness, you must avoid concentrating on just one component. Sometimes people tend to concentrate on what they enjoy the most or do the best. If you really enjoy running but don't like strength training, you may tend to sacrifice the strength training and do more running. That's not bad, but you would be better off doing at least some training for all of the physical fitness components.

Balance comes into play within each component as well. People who are into weightlifting, for example, may concentrate on certain areas of their body and ignore others. The key is to achieve balance among the components of fitness and within each component. You may be the strongest officer in the agency, but if you have ignored your cardiovascular conditioning while concentrating on your strength, you may not be able to catch the suspect to subdue him.

Balance is also important when it comes to injury prevention. Training a muscle while ignoring its antagonist, for example, working the biceps but not the triceps, makes the weaker muscle more susceptible to injury.

PRINCIPLE 7: VARIETY

Variety ties in with balance, recovery, and specificity. Even the most die-hard fitness enthusiasts would get bored if they did the same exercises every day. Vary your routine to reduce the chances of boredom. For example, if you like to swim and have access to a pool, use both swimming and running to develop CVE and keep you excited about exercising. Find different places to train. Explore different weight training routines so that part of your program doesn't become stale.

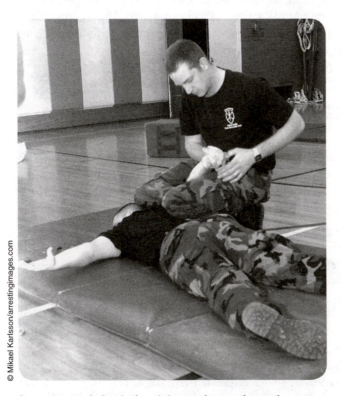

Variety is particularly important for the beginner. In addition to reducing boredom, exposure to multiple activities increases the chances of finding activities you like. And if you like it, you're more apt to stay with it.

As noted in the section on the recovery principle, planning for rest is important. In fact, you can add variety to your program by periodically giving yourself an unexpected and unplanned day off.

Some types of physical activity are better than others at producing results.

PRINCIPLE 8: SPECIFICITY

Specificity in the fitness context means that you get good at what you practice. Running or other cardiovascular activities will not improve your muscular strength, and vice versa. It also means that you will show the greatest improvement in whatever activity you use for training. Running to improve your cardiovascular endurance won't improve your swimming or cycling as much as it will your running ability.

Let's apply this principle to the law enforcement setting and consider strength and defensive tactics training. Getting stronger will help you perform better in a use-of-force situation, but the specific defensive tactics training will further improve that performance.

Balance, variety, and specificity address what *type* of exercise will produce training effects.

PRINCIPLE 9: ADAPTATION

The body adjusts to the effects of training but does so in small increments. Over time, these small increments cause major changes in your body. For example, the increases in muscle mass from strength training don't happen overnight, but one day you will discover that you need a new uniform because the old one doesn't fit the same way anymore. Only by comparing periodic measurements can you truly appreciate the day-to-day adaptations that are occurring. Understanding that fitness is a long-term investment will help avoid frustration and disappointment.

At times during your training, you are going to feel that you have stopped making improvements. This is called plateauing. Don't be discouraged, as this happens to everyone. Stick with your program, and as your body adjusts to the changes that are occurring, you will see continued improvement.

PRINCIPLE 10: INDIVIDUALITY

Each individual will respond somewhat differently to the same training routine. These differences are due to several factors, including heredity, eating and sleeping habits, the environment, illnesses and injuries, level of fitness, and motivation.

The principle of individuality means that some of you are more likely to become more fit in a cardiovascular way than you are to become really strong. Some are more likely to be good runners, others good swimmers, and still others better bikers. And each of you has a different individual potential for how good you can be.

PRINCIPLE 11: MODERATION

Too much of anything can be bad. For best results, you must be dedicated to your program, but temper that dedication with common sense and good judgment. Don't train when you are injured. Also, remember that more is not necessarily better. Too much distance, speed, weight, or time can lead to deterioration rather than development. Moderation in all things, not just physical training, is a good rule for life.

Now that you understand the general application of the principles of fitness, you are ready to apply them to developing training programs for each component of physical fitness. The next four chapters will help you design an individual program for improving your cardiovascular endurance, muscular strength and endurance, flexibility, and anaerobic power.

FITT CHART

This chart will be helpful to you as you train. Feel free to make several copies of this chart.

FITT Chart

Frequency   _____ (number of workouts per week)

Intensity   _____ (how hard you exercise)

Heart rate range   _____ (another measure of how hard you exercise)*

Time   _____ (duration of the workout)

Type   _____ (activity)

*Applies to cardiovascular endurance training program only.

From *Fit for Duty, Second Edition*, by Robert Hoffman and Thomas R. Collingwood, 2005, Champaign, IL: Human Kinetics.

Cardiovascular Endurance

You probably use the word *energy* quite a bit, perhaps in statements such as "I just don't have enough energy" or "I'm going to eat this candy bar to get an energy boost." Most people tend to attribute some nebulous quality to the term, but energy is a very real substance.

Certain foodstuffs stored in the body are released in the presence of oxygen to produce energy. This is called aerobic energy production. Quite simply, the process goes like this (see figure 5.1). We breathe air into our lungs. From there, the oxygen passes into the bloodstream. The better trained our lungs are, the more oxygen is carried by the blood to working muscles. Some things we can control affect how well the blood carries the oxygen. For example, alcohol blocks this ability, diminishing the amount of oxygen that reaches the working muscles.

Next, the oxygen passes from the bloodstream to the muscle, where it combines with stored sugars to produce energy. The amount of sugar stored in the muscle and the efficiency of combining with oxygen are, once again, affected by training.

When the blood leaves the area of the muscle, it removes waste products of the energy production, such as carbon dioxide. The training that improves the various phases of this process also improves cardiovascular endurance (CVE).

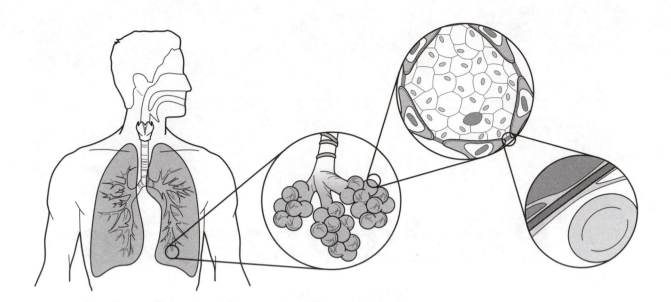

FIGURE 5.1 Aerobic energy production. Air enters the lungs, passes into the bloodstream, and moves to the muscles, where it combines with stored energy. Waste products such as carbon dioxide enter the bloodstream, return to the lungs, and are then exhaled.

WHAT IS CARDIOVASCULAR ENDURANCE?

As you learned in chapter 1, *cardiovascular endurance* is the ability to perform activity that requires the body to combine its energy sources with oxygen. CVE is essential for performing activities that require continuous effort for more than 2 minutes and is important for good health. Law enforcement activities that require cardiovascular endurance include the following:

- Foot pursuits
- Use-of-force situations

Cardiovascular endurance is related to health because it does the following:

- Reduces the risk of heart disease
- Assists in controlling weight, particularly loss of excess body fat
- Helps reduce stress
- Reduces resting blood pressure
- Raises levels of HDL—the good cholesterol
- Helps regulate type II diabetes mellitus
- Helps prevent pulmonary disease
- Lowers the risk for certain cancers, including colon and breast cancers

DESIGNING YOUR CARDIOVASCULAR PROGRAM

Although each of the principles of fitness discussed in chapter 4 applies to cardio-vascular endurance training, some of the applications are quite obvious and won't be discussed here. Instead, we'll concentrate on those that are most important in designing a cardiovascular endurance training program. The program should address these questions:

How often should I exercise?

How hard should I exercise?

How long should I exercise?

What activity should I do?

To answer each of these questions, fill out a copy of the FITT chart on page 56. A summary of the cardiovascular endurance training principles is shown on page 69.

Following are the principles of fitness most applicable to cardiovascular endur-ance training:

- Regularity
- Recovery
- Overload
- Progression
- Variety
- Specificity

Regularity

To improve cardiovascular fitness, you must participate in an appropriate activity, at the necessary intensity and duration, a minimum of three times per training week. More fit people will probably choose to exercise as often as five or six times per training week. However, as you learned in chapter 3, adequate rest is necessary to avoid injury and enhance the positive training effects.

Recovery

Although regularity is important, more is not necessarily better. Without adequate rest, the body's systems and muscles will eventually break down. To apply this principle to cardiovascular training, follow these general rules:

- For those just beginning a training program, alternate days of training with days of rest.
- For more advanced exercisers, avoid training hard on two consecutive days. *Hard* may refer to the intensity or the length of the workout. For example, if

you choose running as your activity for cardiovascular fitness and you train five days a week, you might schedule your training like this:

    Sunday—long, hard

    Monday—short, easy

    Tuesday—short, hard (fast)

    Wednesday—rest

    Thursday—long, easy

    Friday—short, hard

    Saturday—rest

- You should also consider scheduling days of rest after your agency's fitness test, after a road race, or after any all-out effort.

Overload

To understand this principle, consider the stress adaptation syndrome. According to Dr. Hans Selye (1956), a recognized expert on the subject of stress, the body adjusts to the stressors it encounters in everyday life. Each time it makes these adaptations, it becomes better prepared to meet the next stressors—up to a point. If there is insufficient recovery time between each exposure to the stressors, they can overwhelm the body's ability to deal with them. That can cause unnecessary fatigue and injuries. But with sufficient recovery time, the body needs increasingly more difficult challenges to keep improving.

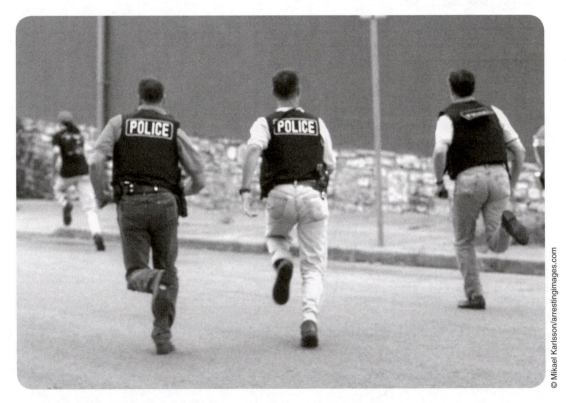

© Mikael Karlsson/arrestingimages.com

Chasing a suspect isn't enough activity to improve your cardiovascular endurance. You must find ways outside of work to improve this area of fitness.

As a law enforcement officer, your day-to-day activities will not give you the cardiovascular endurance necessary for the occasional need to engage in a use-of-force situation or to pursue a suspect. To achieve a training effect, you need to "stress" the cardiovascular system with demands that are greater than your every-day activities. Overload affects two components of FITT: intensity and time.

Intensity

Intensity refers to how hard the exercise should be. You will learn two ways to gauge the intensity of a workout. The first is the target heart rate (THR) method, which uses the heart rate to estimate the intensity of your exercise. The heart rate increases during exercise, as there is a correlation between the heart rate and the overload being placed on the cardiovascular system. To ensure that you are achieving the desired training effect, you must calculate your individual THR for the desired intensity. Because it is an estimate of the work you are doing, and because counting a rapid pulse can be difficult, we recommend that you establish a 20-beat target heart rate range.

To calculate your THR, you will need to know several terms. Recall from chapter 2 that your resting heart rate (RHR) is the number of times your heart beats in a minute while you are at rest. For the most accurate resting pulse, take it first thing in the morning before getting out of bed. That will also give you greater assurance that any variations you notice are due to changes in your body and not to changing conditions.

As your conditioning improves, you should see a gradual decline in your resting heart rate. If you see a sudden increase, it is probably caused by one of two things. You may be overtraining and need a rest, or you may be coming down with a cold or other ailment. You should also know that certain substances, such as caffeine and alcohol, will elevate your heart rate.

Why Is Your RHR Important?

Does lowering your resting heart rate make a difference? It is not uncommon for unfit officers to have an RHR of 80 or even higher. Compared to an officer with an RHR of 60, the unfit officer's heart is beating 28,800 more times every day! Even during the fit officer's cardio-vascular endurance workout, when she might get her heart rate up to 140 beats per minute for 20 minutes, that's only an additional 2,800 beats. CVE training makes the heart muscle stronger so it can push out more blood with each stroke. As a result, the stronger heart can supply the body with sufficient blood using fewer beats. The heart, like any other machine, will last longer when it is stronger and beating fewer times with less wear and tear.

Your maximum heart rate (MHR) is the highest number of beats per minute that your heart is capable of. To estimate MHR, subtract your age from 220. The estimated MHR for a 40-year-old, for example, would be 220 – 40, or 180 beats per minute.

If you have a heart rate monitor, you can measure your maximum heart rate more accurately. Warm up for 10 to 15 minutes by jogging and stretching. Wearing the heart rate monitor, run as fast as you can for a distance of between 200 and

300 meters. The number displayed on the heart rate monitor when you complete the run will be your maximum heart rate.

Let's assume that an officer who could maximize his heart rate at 180 beats per minute has a resting heart rate of 80. Subtracting his RHR from his MHR tells him he has 100 beats "in reserve." That means he can perform activities that require up to 100 additional heartbeats per minute. This is his heart rate reserve (HRR).

The intensity of your workout will be a certain percentage of your HRR. As noted earlier, one of the distinguishing features of CVE training is that it can be sustained over a period of time, so it cannot be an all-out effort. Depending on your fitness level and whether you are planning a hard or easy workout, we recommend that you train between 50 and 80 percent of your HRR.

Now that you know your RHR and MHR and understand that you will choose a percentage of your HRR at which to train, you are ready to calculate your training heart rate range. To do this, you will use what is known as the Karvonen formula. In the example that follows, we take a look at this calculation for our sample officer, choosing a workout intensity of 50 percent.

When taking your pulse during exercise, only count it for 6 seconds and multiply the count by 10. The heart rate drops very quickly when you stop exercising, so for a more accurate estimate, use the 6-second count. In our example, if the officer's training heart rate was lower than 122, he would have to increase his pace to get the desired results. On the other hand, if it was higher than 142, he should slow down his pace.

Example of Calculating Target Heart Rate Range

1. To estimate maximum heart rate (MHR), subtract the individual's age from 220. (Our sample officer is 40.)

$$\begin{array}{r} 220 \\ -\ 40\ \text{age} \\ \hline 180\ \text{MHR} \end{array}$$

2. Subtract the individual's resting heart rate (RHR) from the maximum heart rate to get the heart rate reserve (HRR). (Our sample officer's RHR = 84.)

$$\begin{array}{r} 180 \\ -\ 84\ \text{RHR} \\ \hline 96\ \text{HRR} \end{array}$$

3. Multiply that number by the intensity (the percentage of the maximum heart rate [%MHR] desired).

$$\begin{array}{r} 96 \\ \times 0.50\ \text{MHR} \\ \hline 48 \end{array}$$

4. Find the training heart rate (THR) by adding the resting heart rate to that number.

$$\begin{array}{r} 48 \\ +\ 84\ \text{RHR} \\ \hline 132\ \text{THR} \end{array}$$

5. Set the heart rate range by adding 10 beats below and 10 beats above the training heart rate. Target heart rate range =

$$\begin{array}{r} 132\ \text{THR} \\ \pm\ 10 \\ \hline 122\text{-}142 \end{array}$$

This calculation tells our sample officer that to work at an intensity of 50 percent above his HRR, he should keep his heart rate between 122 and 142 beats per minute.

Use the chart below to calculate your heart rate range for 50, 60, 70, and 80 percent of your HRR. Remember that as your conditioning improves, your resting heart rate will drop, so you will have to recalculate these ranges periodically.

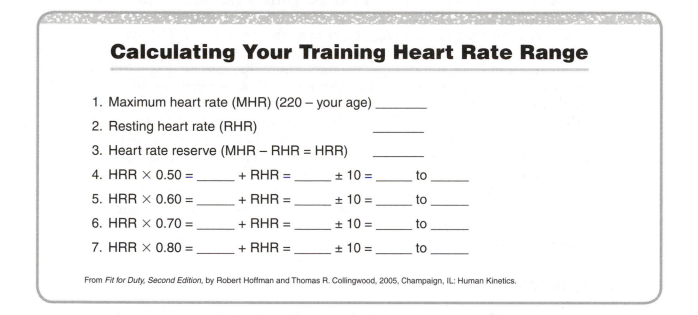

Calculating Your Training Heart Rate Range

1. Maximum heart rate (MHR) (220 – your age) _____

2. Resting heart rate (RHR) _____

3. Heart rate reserve (MHR – RHR = HRR) _____

4. HRR × 0.50 = _____ + RHR = _____ ± 10 = _____ to _____

5. HRR × 0.60 = _____ + RHR = _____ ± 10 = _____ to _____

6. HRR × 0.70 = _____ + RHR = _____ ± 10 = _____ to _____

7. HRR × 0.80 = _____ + RHR = _____ ± 10 = _____ to _____

From *Fit for Duty, Second Edition*, by Robert Hoffman and Thomas R. Collingwood, 2005, Champaign, IL: Human Kinetics.

The other method for estimating the intensity of your workout is the table of perceived exertion. A Swedish psychologist by the name of Borg established that peoples' perceptions of how hard they were working were surprisingly accurate. To use the Borg Perceived Exertion Scale (shown below), simply answer the question, "How does the exercise feel?" The numbers in the left column, when multiplied by 10, will give you an estimate of your heart rate at the perceived level of exertion selected.

6	No exertion at all
7	
8	Extremely light
9	Very light
10	
11	Light
12	
13	Somewhat hard
14	
15	Hard (heavy)
16	
17	Very hard
18	
19	Extremely hard
20	Maximal exertion

Borg RPE scale
© Gunnar Borg, 1970, 1985, 1994, 1998

Time

The other element of overload is time or duration; that is, how long you must keep up the activity to achieve a training effect. As with intensity, duration varies according to your level of conditioning and your goals. It also varies with the type of workout. You can use this variable to alter the results of your workout.

To achieve cardiovascular training, you need to train within your THR range for a minimum of 20 minutes. As your conditioning improves, you may increase this minimum. Generally, as you increase the duration of the exercise, you will have to decrease the intensity to sustain the work for the desired length of time.

Use the results of your fitness assessment to determine your level of conditioning. Here are some guidelines. If you used the 1-mile walk to determine your level of CVE fitness, or ran the 1.5-mile slower than 16 minutes, rate your CVE fitness level as low. You should start with no more than 20 minutes of exercise, if you can last that long. If your time on the 1.5-mile run was between 13 and 16 minutes, consider your fitness level to be average. Your workouts should last between 20 and 60 minutes. For those running the 1.5-mile in under 13 minutes, your fitness level is high to very high. Your workouts are clearly producing results, so keep up the good work!

Progression

The next principle to consider is progression, which also relates to the intensity and time components of FITT. Beginners should expect to see some improvements in about three weeks. For those who are more fit, changes will come about more slowly. Plan to measure your cardiovascular fitness with the 1.5-mile run every six to eight weeks and adjust the intensity and duration accordingly. Remember, to continue to improve, you must increase the overload as your conditioning improves.

You should plan to progress in each of the elements you have read about so far in this training program. When three workouts a week become easy, increase to four. As your conditioning improves, you will find that you can increase the intensity to a higher percentage of your HRR. These improvements will also enable you to increase the time you spend exercising to 25 and then 30 minutes. These changes should be gradual and should continue until you have reached your goals.

You may also reach a level where further improvement is not necessary. If you then continue to work at the same overload, you will maintain your conditioning. Of course, factors such as illness, injury, travel, and aging can all affect this conditioning.

Variety

The last principle to consider when planning your cardiovascular fitness training is variety. You can apply this principle in several ways.

Although the principle of specificity allows you to become good at what you practice, you still might want to vary the activities you use to improve or maintain your cardiovascular fitness. If your goal is general fitness, then combining running, biking, and swimming, for example, will reduce the boredom that may result from doing just one of the activities all the time.

Even if you use only one cardiovascular activity, variety will spice up your training. If you run, choosing different routes, times of the day, and running partners will make the training more interesting.

Specificity and variety relate to the type of activities that can give you a training effect. Activities that will improve your cardiovascular fitness include the following:

Aerobic dance	Rowing
Brisk walking	Running
Cross-country skiing	Stair stepping
Cycling	Swimming
Jogging	In-line skating

The most important consideration in choosing an activity is whether or not you enjoy it.

Specificity

Another factor to consider when developing your training plan is whether you have a specific goal, as opposed to general conditioning. For example, if your agency administers a fitness test, the goal of your cardiovascular training may be to meet the agency's standard. This is where the principle of specificity comes into play. If your agency's test includes a 1.5-mile run, your training plan should include running to improve cardiovascular fitness. Although other types of cardiovascular training, such as swimming, will improve your endurance, they will not prepare you for the 1.5-mile run as well as running will.

For example, an officer with a low fitness level should begin his program with three days of cardiovascular exercise per week. He has decided to choose brisk walking and jogging for his cardiovascular endurance training. His completed cardiovascular training plan would look like this:

Try different activities to keep yourself from getting bored; however, make sure these new activities still help you achieve your specific training goals.

Frequency	Three days per week, with a day of rest between each
Intensity	50 percent
Heart rate range	122-142 beats per minute
Time	20 minutes
Type	Brisk walking and jogging

Remember, although we have used running to demonstrate how to develop a cardiovascular endurance training program, any activity that involves rhythmic movement of large muscle groups for an extended period will produce training effects.

ENVIRONMENTAL GUIDELINES

Environmental conditions can have a significant effect on exercise safety and performance. Someone who trains adapts to training within a certain environment. If that environment changes, an adjustment period is required, normally 30 days, to achieve full acclimatization. Generally, the more fit the individual, the quicker the acclimatization.

Heat and Humidity

Hot weather can cause medical problems and even death. Every part of the country has these conditions at some time of the year. Apply the following hot-weather training guidelines to your fitness program.

Water

- Drink 8 to 10 glasses of water each day to avoid heat stress problems.
- Drink as much water as can be tolerated before, during, and after exercise.
- When considering special athletic drinks for electrolyte replacement, remember that water gets to the muscles more quickly.
- Taking salt tablets is unnecessary. If during hot weather your food tastes more bland than usual or you notice white rings on the underarms of your clothing, pass the salt shaker over your food.
- If your body weight drops by more than 3 percent in one day, drink 2 cups of water to replace each pound of water lost.

Clothing

- Wear clothing that allows maximal evaporation to occur.
- Don't wear rubber or plastic suits.
- Do wear loose clothing made of absorbent materials that wick sweat away from the body.
- Wear light-colored clothing to reflect the heat.
- Don't use oil-based sunscreen.

Training Intensity

- Modify your training until you are partially acclimatized (after 7 to 10 days).
- Don't expect to perform as well as usual.
- Reduce intensity and duration.
- Monitor your heart rate frequently, as it may increase more rapidly than normal.

Monitoring Conditions

- Try to go out during the coolest part of the day, often the early morning.
- Evaluate the heat and humidity conditions to determine whether to exercise and, if so, how strenuously.

Cold

Cold can also cause medical problems and even death. It places a burden on the body for temperature regulation and circulation. Cold stress can affect either peripheral body parts, causing frostbite, or the central core, causing life-threatening hypothermia. Apply the following cold environment training guidelines to your training program.

Water and Food

- Keep your core temperature up.
- Drink plenty of fluids. Dehydration is also a problem in cold weather.
- Avoid drinking alcohol.
- Eat plenty of carbohydrate. Because cold conditions raise the body's metabolism, fuel burns up more quickly.

Clothing

- Dress warmly for protection, yet avoid sweating.
- Avoid sweating by dressing in removable, loose-fitting layers.
- Wear fabrics that draw moisture away from the body.
- Wear an outer layer that is wind resistant.
- Wear a hat and something to cover your neck.
- Wear mittens rather than gloves, as the fingers stay warmer when in contact with each other.

Training Intensity

- Warm up well before exercising and cool down indoors.
- Lower your exercise intensity.
- Keep moving.

Monitoring Conditions

- Try to go out during the warmest part of the day, often the early afternoon.
- Evaluate the cold conditions to determine whether to exercise and, if so, how strenuously.

Altitude

At higher elevations, there is less oxygen in the air, so exercisers must work harder to maintain a given level of activity. Altitude starts to have a major effect on the body between 5,000 and 7,000 feet. The body adapts to a higher altitude by developing more red blood cells so more of the limited oxygen can be distributed. Until that acclimatization occurs, any workload will be more demanding, so workout intensity should be decreased.

The major problem caused by altitude is altitude sickness, a condition that occurs when one is physically active at an altitude one hasn't adapted to yet. Cold-weather problems may also occur at higher altitudes. Apply the following altitude training guidelines to your fitness program.

Water—Drink plenty of water before, during, and after exercise.

Clothing—Wear the same clothing as for cold weather.

Training intensity—Generally, intensity needs to be lowered.

Monitoring conditions—Keep track of wind chill.

Pollution

Pollution poses a similar problem to that of altitude: There is not enough oxygen in the air because of competing pollutants. This lack of oxygen makes exercise more difficult, and breathing in the pollutants is potentially harmful as well. Pollution also makes exercising uncomfortable because of eye, nose, and lung irritation. Three main pollutants cause respiratory stress:

- Ozone, which reduces cardiovascular endurance
- Sulfur dioxide, which can narrow the airways and make breathing more difficult, especially for asthmatics
- Carbon monoxide, which competes with oxygen for placement on red blood cells

Apply the following pollution training guidelines to your fitness program.

Time of day—Don't schedule exercise between 7 and 10 a.m. and 4 and 7 p.m., as pollution levels tend to be higher during peak traffic periods.

Place—Attempt to exercise in a location with low pollution.

Reduce exposure—As the effects of pollution accumulate over time, limit outdoor exercise if possible.

WARMING UP AND COOLING DOWN

Although by now you may have a pretty good idea of what the warm-up and cool-down entail, here's a brief description of what they are and how they are accomplished.

Warm up before physical activity to prepare the muscles for the more vigorous activity to follow. Warming up provides a transition as the body moves from rest to activity. It helps prevent injury and enhances performance. The warm-up has two parts: light movement followed by static stretches (you will learn about these stretches in chapter 7). Start with some easy, rhythmic movements to warm the muscles. A good rule of thumb is to do enough easy running in place or jumping jacks to develop a light sweat before stretching. The static stretching part of the warm-up should concentrate on the muscles to be used in the activity to follow.

Many people who wouldn't consider exercising without warming up first completely ignore the cool-down. Yet easy movement and static stretching at the end of a workout may be just as important as warming up. One benefit of cooling down seems to be reduced muscle soreness. And just as the warm-up serves as a transition from rest to activity, the cool-down provides a gradual transition back to rest.

These warm-up and cool-down guidelines are not just important for cardiovascular training but should be applied to all the exercise routines.

Summary of Cardiovascular Endurance Training Principles

The following summarizes the information you need to design your cardiovascular endurance training plan using the FITT acronym.

Factor	Low fitness	Average fitness	High fitness
Frequency	3 days/week	3-5 days/week	3-7 days/week
Intensity	50-60 percent	50-70 percent	50-80 percent
Time	20 minutes	20-60 minutes	>30 minutes
Type	Walk, swim, cycle	Previous types plus run, group exercise, row, aerobic dance	Previous types plus cross-country skiing, step aerobics

Resistance Strength Training

When most people think about making muscles bigger and stronger, they picture a weight room with bars, weights, benches, and machines. Traditionally, this type of training was referred to as *weight* or *strength* training. However, there are other ways to build strength, and for some performers, muscular endurance is more important than muscular strength. For purposes of this chapter, we will call this type of training *resistance* training, which encompasses the traditional weight training with free weights as well as with machines, resistance bands, a partner, and calisthenics.

When you hear the term *resistance training*, do you picture a Ron Coleman type lifting huge weights in the gym? For those who have never participated in a resistance training program, that would be a likely response and would also likely be quite intimidating. But even Ron went into the gym for the first time one day, and he didn't get that body overnight. Not that the goal of your resistance training program needs to be, or should be, that type of physique. In fact, unless you chose your parents very carefully, it probably isn't possible.

Muscular strength and endurance are perhaps the most important components of physical fitness for law enforcement officers. Not only do several essential job functions require strength and endurance, but stronger officers are less likely to get injured in the performance of duty. Also, when injuries do occur, officers with higher levels of muscular fitness recover more quickly.

This chapter will give you the information you need to design a program to improve both your strength and muscular endurance and help improve your performance. You will also learn various ways to develop muscular strength and endurance, including techniques such as resistance bands, which do not require expensive equipment. We will also discuss calisthenics and partner-resisted exercises.

WHAT ARE MUSCULAR STRENGTH AND MUSCULAR ENDURANCE?

We all have a pretty good idea of what the term *strength* means; however, we sometimes confuse muscular strength with muscular endurance. In its purest sense, strength is a muscle's ability to generate maximum force. The greatest resistance a muscle can overcome through its range of motion one time is called one-repetition maximum (1RM). Resistance is generally some amount of weight that you are lifting or pushing, for example, a set of dumbbells. But it could also be your own body weight while doing a push-up or pull-up or the opposition presented by a partner while doing partner-resisted exercises.

Muscular endurance is the muscle's ability to overcome a given resistance for multiple repetitions or for an extended time without too much fatigue. For example, doing a push-up requires a certain amount of strength in the chest, shoulders, and triceps. Doing 30 push-ups requires the same amount of strength but also requires muscular endurance. Here are some additional terms you will need to know.

full range of motion—Moving the muscle from a fully extended position to complete flexion.

grip—Refers to how you hold the bar or dumbbell. An overhand grip means the palm is facing away from the body, whereas for an underhand grip, the palm is toward the body. For safety, you should always use a positive or closed grip with the thumb wrapped around the bar or handle.

momentary muscle failure—Occurs when you are no longer able to perform a correct repetition.

dumbbell—A type of free weight. It is configured to be held in one hand and comes in various weights.

free weights—What often comes to mind when picturing traditional strength training. Free weights include the straight bar, usually weighing 45 pounds. You would normally slip weight plates on either end of the bar to create the desired resistance. The plates come in various weights: 5, 10, 25, 35, and 45 pounds. For safety, you should use collars to hold the plates on the bar.

weight machines—Control all aspects of the range of motion and movement for an exercise. They have standard weight plates that allow less variation of resistance than free weights.

repetition—The performance of an exercise from the starting position through the full range of motion and back to the start. For example, a repetition of the biceps curl using free weights would start with the arms fully extended, with the weight in front of the quadriceps. To begin the exercise, you would raise the weight by bending your arms at the elbows. After reaching full flexion, you would return the weight to the starting position by fully extending your arms to lower the weight. This constitutes a repetition.

set—A predetermined number of repetitions performed consecutively. The number of repetitions is determined by the goal of the workout; that is, to build strength (1 to 6 reps), gain endurance (15 to 20 reps), or develop a combination (8 to 12 reps). New exercisers should begin with one set and build up to three. More advanced exercisers may start with three sets and build up to five.

Resistance training is specific to the type of contraction the muscle performs. Three types of contraction exist: isometric, isotonic, and isokinetic.

Isometric Contractions

Isometric (or static) contractions involve the muscle contracting against an immovable and unvarying resistance. For example, standing in an open doorway and pushing out against the doorjambs would be an isometric contraction. These contractions strengthen the muscle only at the angle at which the exercise is performed, not through the entire range of motion. Isometric exercises should not be done by those with cardiac conditions, as such exercises elevate the blood pressure.

Isotonic Contractions

Isotonic contractions occur when the muscle goes through two phases of contraction: concentric and eccentric.

- During the concentric phase of movement, the muscle shortens. Sometimes this is called positive work. Figure 6.1a shows the concentric phase as the weight is lifted in an arm curl.

- During the eccentric phase of movement, the muscle lengthens back to normal. Sometimes this is called negative work. Figure 6.1b shows the eccentric phase as the weight is lowered in an arm curl.

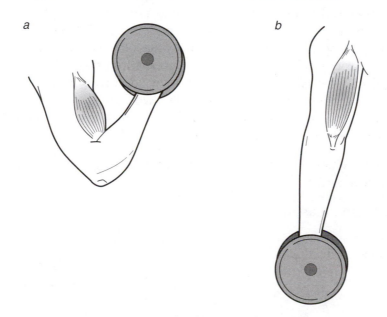

FIGURE 6.1   Arm curl: *(a)* concentric contraction and *(b)* eccentric contraction.

Most resistance training programs (whether free weight, machine, or calisthenics) are isotonic training programs because you live in an isotonic world. Daily use of muscles, whether at work, play, or sport, requires isotonic contractions.

Isokinetic Contractions

Isokinetic contractions occur when the speed of contraction is controlled and the resistance accommodates to the force applied. Isokinetic contractions are only concentric. Special equipment is required to produce isokinetic contractions.

DEVELOPING MUSCULAR STRENGTH

Muscle strength (force) depends primarily on two factors:

- **Size.** The larger the cross-sectional size of the muscle, the greater the force that can be generated.
- **Fiber recruitment.** Muscles are made up of bundles of fibers. When a muscle contracts, only a percentage of the fibers contract at one time. The percentage is based on how much effort is necessary to overcome the resistance. Consequently, the more fibers that are contracting, the greater the force generated.

Two other factors that affect muscle development are gender and the type of muscle fibers present.

- **Gender.** Men tend to accommodate to resistance training by increasing size, women by increasing fiber recruitment. The reason is that men have more testosterone (a male sex hormone) than women, and testosterone helps build tissue.
- **Type of muscle fibers.** We have two basic types of muscle fibers. Slow-twitch fibers appear red under a microscope and are better adapted for activities involving the use of oxygen to produce energy. Long-distance runners tend to have higher percentages of this type of fiber. The other type is fast-twitch fibers. They appear white under a microscope and respond better to resistance training than slow-twitch fibers do. Heredity determines how much of each fiber type we have, which explains why two people may train identically but one develops more strength. Specific training improves the functional ability of both types of fibers.

Law enforcement activities that require muscular strength and endurance (MSE) include the following:

Use-of-force situations

Climbing

Lifting and carrying

Dragging

Pushing

Pulling

Muscular strength and endurance are related to health because they do the following:

    Help prevent injury

    Delay the onset of osteoporosis

    Help prevent low back pain

DESIGNING YOUR RESISTANCE TRAINING PROGRAM

This section will discuss the principles of training most pertinent to resistance training. These principles apply to all forms of resistance training, but weight training will be used as the example here. As you design your program, you will answer the questions of how often, how hard, how long, and what activities will produce a training effect. Fill out a copy of the FITT chart on page 56 to help you answer these questions. A summary of the resistance training principles is shown on page 93. The following principles of exercise are especially important to resistance training:

    Overload

    Progression

    Specificity

    Regularity

    Recovery

    Balance

    Variety

Keep in mind that any activity you use to overcome resistance will produce a training effect if it conforms to these principles. The activity may be lifting weight using free weights or machines, stretching resistance bands, moving your own body weight using calisthenics, or pushing/pulling your partner using partner-resisted exercises.

Overload

For a muscle to increase in strength or endurance, you must place a higher workload on the muscle than is provided by your normal daily activity. Workload can be defined in terms of resistance (pounds lifted), the number of sets, and the number of repetitions in each set of repeated exercises. Over time, with regular workouts, the accumulated infinitesimal increases in muscle size become visible, and you can see musculature develop. Look at the increase in muscle size shown in figure 6.2. Overload relates to two components of FITT: intensity and time (duration).

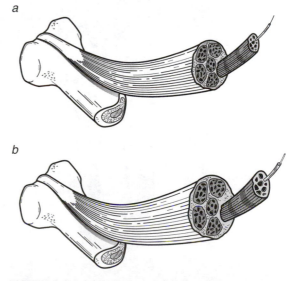

a

b

FIGURE 6.2 *(a)* Before and *(b)* after long-term training. Notice how the size of the muscle fibers has increased.

Intensity

One of the variables in resistance training is how much weight will be lifted for each exercise. One method often used for determining intensity is to work with percentages of the most weight you can lift in one all-out effort, or your one-repetition maximum. The procedure is as follows:

- **Select exercises.** Select the exercises for your program. Your routine should exercise the major muscle groups necessary for basic physical movement and physical performance. These groups are shown in figure 6.3.
- **Determine the 1RM for each exercise.** For each exercise, start with a weight you can easily lift one time. Add weight until you have determined the most weight you can lift in one try. This is your 1RM. You can estimate the 1RM of an exercise using the same testing process options described for the 1RM bench press test in chapter 3.

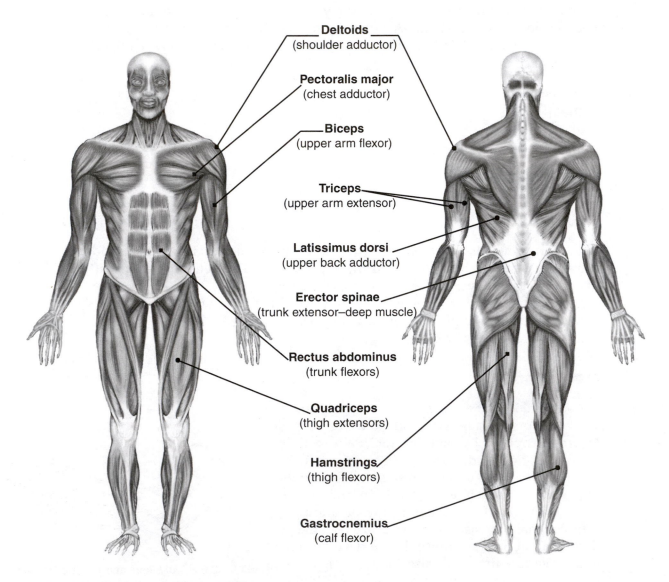

Deltoids
(shoulder adductor)

Pectoralis major
(chest adductor)

Biceps
(upper arm flexor)

Triceps
(upper arm extensor)

Latissimus dorsi
(upper back adductor)

Erector spinae
(trunk extensor–deep muscle)

Rectus abdominus
(trunk flexors)

Quadriceps
(thigh extensors)

Hamstrings
(thigh flexors)

Gastrocnemius
(calf flexor)

FIGURE 6.3   Muscle groups used to exercise.

Depending on whether you are trying to develop strength, endurance, or a combination of the two, the percentage of 1RM you work with will vary from 40 to 100 percent.

- If the goal is muscular strength, use high resistance (80 to 100 percent of 1RM).
- If the goal is muscular endurance, use low resistance (40 to 60 percent of 1RM).
- If the goal is a combination of strength and endurance, use medium resistance (60 to 80 percent of 1RM).

You can use the Resistance Training Planning Form below to design your training plan. If you choose to establish your 1RM for each exercise, enter it in the second column. For sit-ups and back extensions, enter the number of repetitions performed in 1 minute. Enter your starting weight (40 to 80 percent of 1RM) in the third column for the exercises using weights and 50 percent of the 1-minute maximum for sit-ups and back extensions.

Resistance Training Planning Form

Muscle group	1RM or estimated 1RM	Percent training weight	Week 1 reps/sets	Week 2 reps/sets	Week 3 reps/sets	Week 4 reps/sets
Leg press/ squats	____	____	__ __	__ __	__ __	__ __
Bench press	____	____	__ __	__ __	__ __	__ __
Leg flexion	____	____	__ __	__ __	__ __	__ __
Bent rowing/ pull-down	____	____	__ __	__ __	__ __	__ __
Shoulder press	____	____	__ __	__ __	__ __	__ __
Sit-ups/ abdominal curl	____	____	__ __	__ __	__ __	__ __
Trunk lifts/ back extension	____	____	__ __	__ __	__ __	__ __
Calf raises	____	____	__ __	__ __	__ __	__ __
Biceps curl	____	____	__ __	__ __	__ __	__ __
Triceps extension	____	____	__ __	__ __	__ __	__ __

From *Fit for Duty, Second Edition*, by Robert Hoffman and Thomas R. Collingwood, 2005, Champaign, IL: Human Kinetics.

Time or Duration

Although you won't actually be timing your resistance workouts as you will your cardiovascular endurance workouts, we will use the term *time* for consistency. The equivalent of time for resistance training is how many repetitions and sets you do of each exercise.

- For increasing strength, do 1 to 6 reps per set.
- For increasing endurance, do 15 to 20 reps per set.
- For increasing both strength and endurance, do 8 to 12 reps per set.

Most officers we have worked with over the years have stated "toning up" as the goal of their resistance training program. An endurance workout of 15 to 20 reps best supports this goal; however, many beginners find that number of reps to be a bit daunting. Therefore, even if toning is your long-range goal, you may consider starting with workouts of 8 to 12 reps until you develop the exercise habit. Later, you can increase the number of reps to 15 to 20. To determine the starting weights for your program, determine 60 to 80 percent of your 1RM for each exercise. Start with 60 percent of your 1RM and see if you can do 8 reps correctly. If not, reduce the weight until you can. If you can do 12 reps correctly, increase the weight until you reach a weight at which 8 to 11 reps can be done correctly before reaching muscle failure—when you can no longer perform a correct repetition of the exercise. Use that weight until you can do 12 reps correctly. For sit-ups and trunk lifts (back extensions), divide the number done in 1 minute in half to get the number of training repetitions.

Beginners should start with one set of each exercise. To build both strength and endurance, do 8 to 12 reps per set.

Note of Caution

If you are a beginner, trying to establish a 1RM may not be safe. We recommend that beginners experiment to find a starting resistance with which you can perform between 8 and 12 correct repetitions. Once you can do 12 good reps, increase the resistance by 5 to 25 percent.

Progression

As a muscle adjusts to a new workload, the workload must be increased again to continue seeing improvement. For each exercise, increase the weight by 5 to 25 percent once 12 reps can be done correctly. Between 8 and 11 reps should be possible with the new weight. For sit-ups and trunk lifts, retest every four weeks.

Some experts suggest that you limit increases to 5 percent. This is virtually impossible for low-end performers. For example, someone who has a starting weight of 20 pounds for the biceps curl builds up to be able to perform 12 correct reps. Adding 5 percent would raise the resistance to 21 pounds—not very practical. Adding 25 percent would mean using 25 pounds. If this individual were only able to perform 6 correct reps with 25 pounds, he could finish the set with the 20-pound weight.

Gradually work up to and maintain three sets of the exercises for each training session. If you have the time and motivation, you can do up to five sets; however, research indicates that the additional training effect per set diminishes considerably after the third set.

Plan to train at least three days per week. (Although training three days per week may seem to be the same as training every other day, the latter actually results in 17 percent more training effect and caloric expenditure.) As your conditioning improves, you may decide to alter parts of your training plan. You may find that your schedule precludes training any more often than three times a week but that you can complete the workout with a higher percentage of your 1RM. You should also gradually increase the number of sets until you reach three. As you increase the number of sets, you may have to cut back on the amount of weight you are lifting, especially in the last set. That's okay because as your muscles adapt to the new overload, you will eventually be able to complete three sets with the heavier weight.

Specificity

Training is specific to the muscle, the contraction movement, the joint angle, the apparatus or equipment used, and the demand placed on the muscle. Upper body training will not increase lower body strength, and vice versa. Select a series of exercises to work a wide range of muscle groups. Plan to train all 10 muscle groups shown in figure 6.3. You can increase muscular strength and endurance by employing the principle of specificity. Several years ago, we conducted a push-up improvement study in response to concerns from the field that women couldn't develop adequate upper body muscular endurance. By training three times a week for 10 to 15 minutes per session, the women in the study improved from an average of 9.3 to 23.7 push-ups. The pretest average was largely influenced by a 43-year-old woman, a regular in the weight room, who did 35 push-ups. We expected her to show the least improvement because she already had a high level of upper body muscular endurance. However, after practicing for six weeks, she became very good at doing push-ups and did 63 in the posttest! Specificity does matter.

Regularity

Resistance training must be consistent over time. Strength cannot be saved up; it must be maintained constantly with regular resistance training. Recent evidence indicates that strength gains may take place with as few as two training sessions per week. Fitter people may choose to train more often. Although it might take several weeks of inactivity to notice a detraining effect, the muscles actually start losing strength after 96 hours.

Recovery

Although regular exercise is crucial, the same muscle should not be worked to exhaustion on consecutive days. The muscle needs time to recover before being worked again. As a rule of thumb, rest for at least 48 hours and no more than 96 hours between hard workouts for the same muscle groups. To apply this principle to resistance training, consider the following guidelines:

- Those just beginning a training program should alternate days of training with days of rest.

- More advanced exercisers may train on consecutive days but should avoid working the same muscle group on two consecutive days. Two examples of how more advanced exercisers can apply the principle of recovery are shown below.

Sample Resistance Training Schedules for More Advanced Exercisers

Alternate days	Alternate body parts
Sunday—rest	Sunday—rest
Monday—all body parts	Monday—upper body
Tuesday—rest	Tuesday—lower body
Wednesday—all body parts	Wednesday—rest
Thursday—rest	Thursday—upper body
Friday—all body parts	Friday—lower body
Saturday—rest	Saturday—rest

You should also consider scheduling days of rest before and after your agency's fitness test or before and after any all-out effort. If you have not been working out on a regular basis, begin by training every other day.

Balance

All muscles should be exercised regularly to avoid an imbalance between muscles and to develop overall body strength and endurance. Muscular strength imbalances can cause injuries. For example, a strength and conditioning coach for a national powerhouse college football program identified that strength imbalances between the quads and hamstrings were resulting in hamstring pulls. After he implemented a team rule that prohibited athletes from practicing if the strength levels of those muscle groups were not within 10 percent of each other, the team went more than 25 years without a pulled hamstring. Resistance training can be applied to all muscles that provide movement. Very specific routines can be developed to increase muscle strength and performance in particular ways.

Muscle groups and the free weight and exercise machine exercises that work them are shown on the following page. (The free weight exercises are then described in detail on pages 82-86.) Many different types of machines are available for each exercise. Although they are similar, you should refer to the instructional manual for each machine to ensure proper execution. If you do not have access to the manual, get some instruction and supervision from someone with more experience.

Weight Training Exercises

Muscle group	Free weights	Exercise machines	Recommendations and cautions
Gastrocnemius	Heel raises with weight on back	Calf raises	Use a 2-inch lift or step. Do 10 reps with toes pointed straight ahead, 10 with toes pointed out, and 10 with toes pointed in.
Hamstrings	Leg flexion	Leg flexion	Resistance should be enough that it takes 2 seconds to raise the leg, 4 seconds to lower it.
Quadriceps	Half knee bends (or squats) with weight on back	Leg press or leg extensions	For free weights, lower buttocks until thigh is parallel with ground. Keep movement smooth without any bouncing.
Abdominals	Sit-ups	Abdominal curl machine	For sit-ups, keep legs bent at 90-degree angle. Don't lift buttocks off the ground.
Latissimus dorsi	Bent rowing	Pull-down	Pull bar to chest, not stomach.
Pectorals	Bench press	Bench press	Do not arch back.
Erector spinae	Trunk lifts	Back extension machine	Not recommended for those with back problems.
Deltoids	Military press	Seated shoulder press	For free weights, alternate lowering weight in front of and behind head.
Biceps	Curls	Curls	Keep back straight.
Triceps	Triceps extension	Triceps extension	With free weights, this exercise also can be done lying on a bench.

Free Weight Exercises

The following exercise descriptions correspond to the exercises listed in Weight Training Exercises on page 81. Only the free weight exercises are illustrated here because the wide variety of exercise machines available would make it difficult to illustrate every possible variation. (Also, weight machines put your body in the correct position for a given lift. When using machines, be sure to read the instructions on the side of the machine for each exercise.)

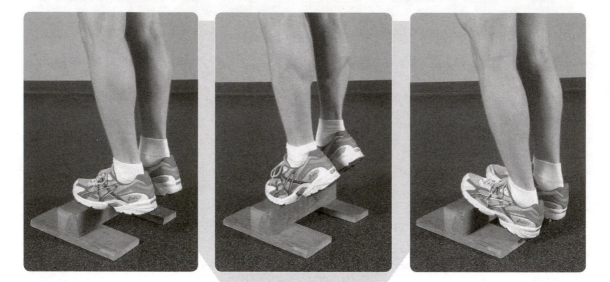

Heel Raises

Stand on an elevated, stable surface such as a step or a 2-inch lift. Place your feet hip-width apart with the balls of both feet near the front of the step so your heels are hanging over the edge. You may vary the position of your feet from pointing straight ahead to pointing slightly outward or inward. Keep your torso erect and your knees straight. Slowly raise your heels as high as possible. Pause for 2 seconds. Allow only your calves to do the work. Exhale as you ascend. While counting to four, lower your heels to a full stretch without pain. Do not move your torso or flex your knees. Inhale as you descend. If performing this exercise with just your body weight is too easy, add some resistance by holding a dumbbell in each hand or placing a straight bar across your shoulders. As your calves become stronger, you should increase the resistance.

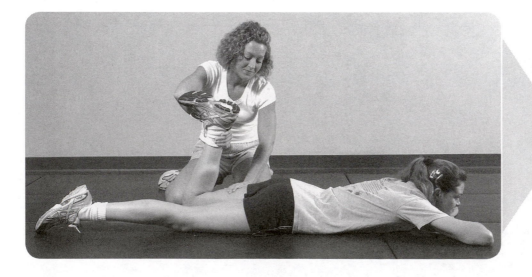

Leg Flexion

You'll need a partner for this exercise. Lie face down with your legs extended. Flex one leg against your partner's resistance until your heel is as close to your buttocks as possible. Next, resist your partner's efforts as she returns your leg to the starting position. Repeat this exercise with the other leg.

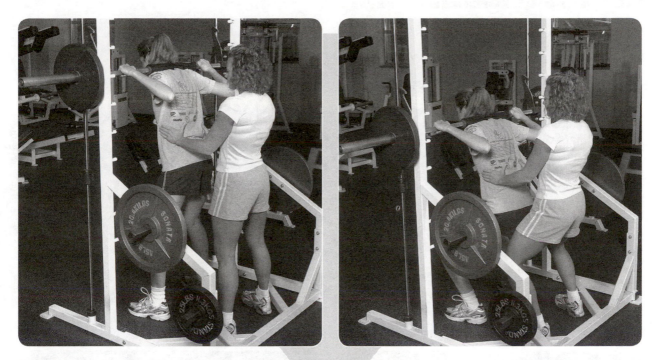

Half Knee Bends (or Squats) With Weight on Back

You'll need a spotter for this exercise. Grasp a straight bar with an overhand grip, your hands slightly wider than shoulder-width apart, and place the bar on your shoulders at the base of your neck. Keep your torso and hips directly under the bar with your chest out, your shoulders back, and your head up. Your feet should be flat on the floor, slightly more than shoulder-width apart. The spotter should stand directly behind you, keeping her back flat and knees flexed. Squat down to a count of two, inhaling as you descend. Avoid leaning forward, and keep your feet flat on the floor with your knees in line with your feet. Squat until the backs of your thighs are parallel with the floor. Begin the upward movement with your legs first, keeping your head up and chest out. Straighten your hips and knees, and exhale as you count to four.

Sit-Ups and Crunches

Crunches are preferred if you have a lower back problem or if you can not do a regular sit-up. (For instructions on how to perform sit-ups, please see chapter 3, page 42.) Lie with your back and feet flat on the floor and your knees flexed to 90 degrees. Fold your arms across your chest. Curl your chin to your chest first and then raise your shoulders and upper back to a 30- to 45-degree angle, exhaling as you sit up. If you can't perform a sit-up this way, anchor your feet under a couch or have a partner hold them. Pause in the up position and then slowly return to the starting position, inhaling as you move down. Keep your chin to your chest until your shoulders touch the mat, and then lower your head. Pause in this position before beginning another repetition. As it gets easier, hold a weight on your chest.

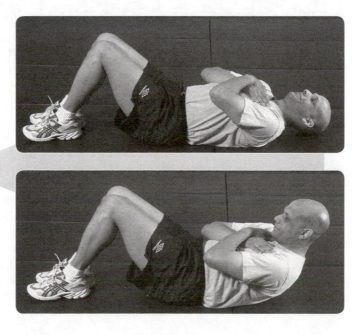

(continued)

Free Weight Exercises *(continued)*

Bent Rowing

Use an overhand grip with your hands at least shoulder-width apart and your shoulders higher than your hips. Your lower back should be flat, your elbows straight, your head facing forward, and your knees slightly flexed. Slowly pull the bar straight up and pause momentarily before it touches your chest. Keep your torso rigid, and exhale as the bar nears your chest. Inhale as you slowly lower the bar straight down, taking care not to bounce or jerk the bar at the bottom. Do not allow the bar to touch the floor until the set is complete.

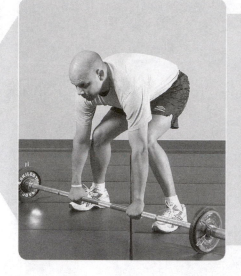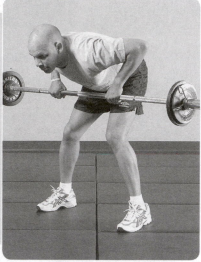

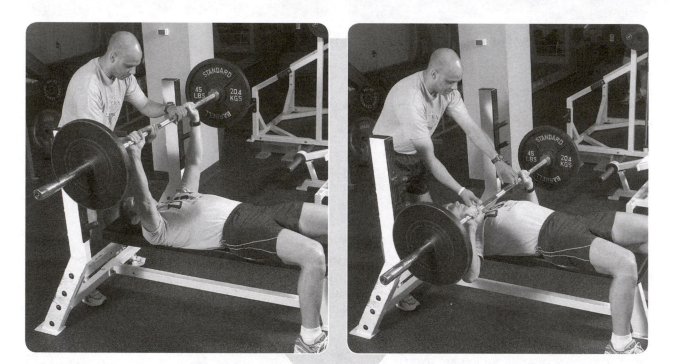

Bench Press

You'll need a spotter for this exercise. Use an overhand grip with your hands at least shoulder-width apart. Position your body so that you have four points of contact—your head, shoulders, and buttocks on the bench and your feet on the floor. The spotter should position his feet 2 to 6 inches from the bench and use an alternate grip inside your hands. Signal the spotter to assist you in moving the bar off the supports. Push the bar to a straight-elbow position over your chest. The spotter should assist with moving the bar off the supports and should guide the bar to the straight-elbow position. Throughout the rest of the exercise, the spotter's hands should closely follow the bar's movement, ready to assist if necessary. Inhale as you slowly lower the bar to your chest. Keep your wrists straight and directly above your elbows. Exhale as you push the bar upward under control. Your elbows should extend evenly, and your wrists should be directly above your elbows. Pause at the straight-elbow position.

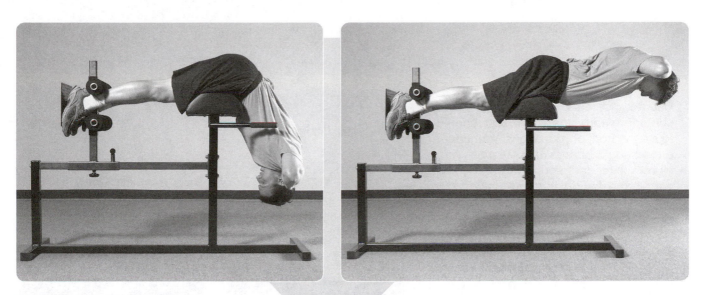

Trunk Lifts

Lie face down on a hyperextension bench with your knees level with your hips. The pads should be in contact with your hips and the backs of your ankles. Lower your torso to form a 90-degree angle at the hips. Place your hands on the sides of your head or cross them at your chest. You can add resistance by holding a weight plate. Raise your trunk until your torso is parallel with the floor. Your head should face forward and your thighs and shoulders should form a straight line. Exhale throughout the upward movement. Inhale as you slowly lower your upper body to the starting position.

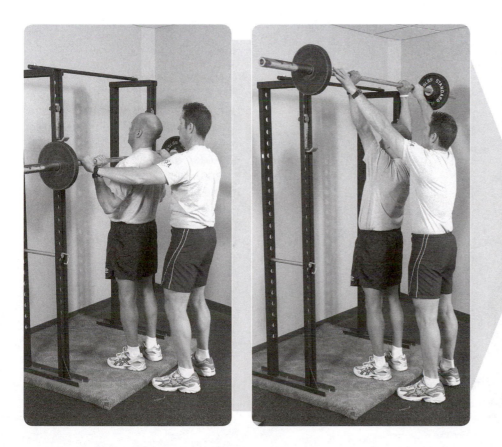

Military Press

Use an overhand grip with your hands at least shoulder-width apart. Keep your head upright and facing forward, and keep your elbows under the bar with your wrists extended. The bar should rest in your hands and on your chest. A spotter should stand directly behind you, as close as possible, with feet shoulder-width apart. Throughout the rest of the exercise, the spotter's hands should closely follow the bar. Push the bar straight up while keeping your back flat and erect. Exhale through the sticking point and pause at the top of the movement. Lower the bar slowly while inhaling. Do not bounce the bar off your upper chest.

(continued)

Free Weight Exercises (continued)

Biceps Curls

Use an underhand grip with your hands shoulder-width apart. The bar should touch the front of your thighs. Your upper arms should be against your ribs, your elbows extended, your torso erect, and your head facing forward. Keep your upper arms stationary and your elbows close to your body as you curl the bar to your shoulders. Be careful not to rock, jerk, or swing your body as you lift. Exhale as the bar nears your shoulders. Inhale during the downward movement, lowering the bar slowly to your thighs. Keep your elbows close to your sides and extend your arms completely.

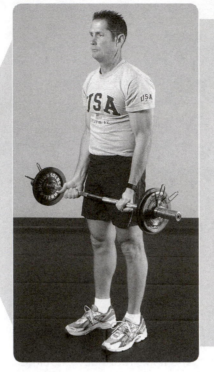
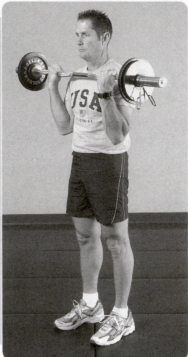

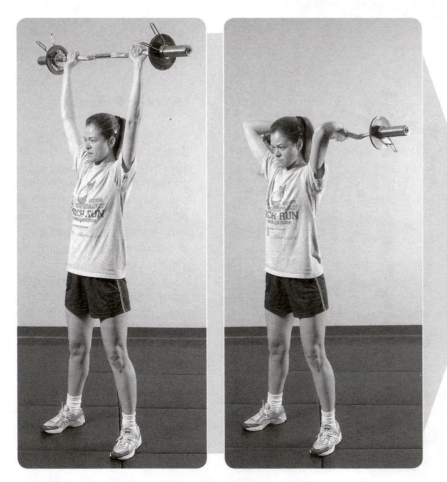

Triceps Extension

Use an overhand grip with your hands 6 inches apart. Keep your torso erect, your head facing forward, your feet shoulder-width apart, and your fully extended elbows close to your ears. Inhale as you lower the bar behind your head to the top of your shoulders. Keep your elbows pointed up, and control the downward movement of the bar. Then push the bar until your elbows are again fully extended. Keep your elbows back and close to your ears. Exhale as the bar passes through the sticking point.

Variety

As with any training, doing the same routine over and over again will get boring. Evidence also suggests that muscles may be resistant to continued growth if you always use the same routine. You can obtain a strength and endurance training effect in many ways. As you become more experienced, look for new exercises to train the same muscle groups. If you have access to several different types of equipment, try them. For an occasional change of pace, consider doing the calisthenics routine described later in this chapter. Pack your resistance bands when you are taking a trip. Using free weights, machines, or resistance bands, or even pushing against the resistance of a partner, can help you achieve the desired effect.

RESISTANCE TRAINING TIPS

Several lessons that are not covered by the principles of exercise will make your training safer and more effective.

1. Warm up with calisthenics and stretching for 3 to 5 minutes before doing a resistance workout. Part of the warm-up can consist of lifting lighter weights than you normally train with.

2. Start with the largest muscle groups and work down to the smallest. Small muscles are generally involved at least as stabilizers when you exercise the large muscles. If you exhaust them before you finish training the larger muscles, you will be unable to get as much work done with the larger muscles. If you plan to exercise all the major muscle groups in the same workout, a recommended sequence would be legs, back, chest, shoulders, arms, and neck. The abdominals can be exercised every day if you desire.

3. Exercise the muscles through the full range of motion (FROM). Before performing an exercise for the first time, move the body part to be exercised as far as it can go from the starting position to full extension and back again. This is the full range of motion of that muscle for that exercise. Start from the stretched position, move to the contracted position, and then return to the stretched position. For maximum strength gains, do each exercise through the FROM.

4. Control the weight, and avoid fast and jerky movements. The purpose of this rule is to avoid injury while getting the maximum benefit from each repetition. Lift the weight with a smooth, controlled motion. Do not "throw" the weight. Counting to two as you lift the weight will help you get the right speed of movement. Lower the weight slowly, counting to four, because the negative phase should take about twice as long as the positive phase. There are two reasons for this. First, the same muscles are used to lower the weight as to lift it. Second, you can lower much more weight than you can lift, so there is potential for more strength gain in the negative phase. If you are working with a partner, include some negative work in each session. Have your partner help you lift a weight that you can't lift by yourself, and then slowly lower it. Repeat until you can no longer safely control the weight's descent. Or, at the end of a regular set of an exercise when you can no longer lift a weight by yourself, have your partner help you back to the starting position, and then you lower the weight. Repeat until you can no longer safely control the weight's descent.

5. Exercise a muscle to momentary failure. A muscle consists of thousands of individual fibers. For each bout of work, only the number of fibers that are required to accomplish the work are recruited for the job. To ensure maximum participation of the fibers, you need to work the muscle to exhaustion.

6. Rest between each set of exercises. For endurance exercises, rest for 1.5 to 2 minutes; for strength exercises, rest for 3 to 5 minutes; for both combined, rest for 30 to 60 seconds.

7. Practice proper form. Most people find it more comfortable to exhale while lifting the weight and inhale while lowering the weight. Do not hold your breath or hyperventilate. If training with free weights, keep the weights close to your body.

8. Whenever possible, work with a partner. This has three advantages. One is that you are more likely to push yourself when someone is there with you. Another is that you can more easily accomplish negative work. Finally, it is safer to work with a partner. You and your partner should know how to spot for each other. Spotters are essential for free weight lifters and provide the following benefits:

   • Ensure that weights don't fall on the lifter or others
   • Give the lifter confidence to try heavier weights or do additional repetitions
   • Offer motivation
   • Assist as the lifter reaches muscle failure

   Spotters should have the following qualities:
   • Enough strength to assist with the weights being lifted
   • Knowledge about where to stand and how to grip the bar
   • Alertness for signs of trouble
   • Willingness to encourage the lifter to make a maximum effort and to maintain correct form

   For spotting to work, the lifter must communicate with the spotter. The lifter must tell the spotter how many reps he plans to attempt and during what rep he is likely to need help.

RESISTANCE BANDS

Many officers have found using resistance bands to be an effective, convenient, and economical approach to resistance training. You can replicate any exercise you can perform with free weights or machines using resistance bands. Resistance band sets normally include an instruction booklet with diagrams. If you do not have one, visualize the exercise you want to perform, and imitate how you would do it with weights.

A set of resistance bands provides added flexibility to your training. You can use them to exercise in the comfort of your home, and they are easily transportable to help you stay in your routine when traveling. On pleasant days when you may not feel like being in the gym, take your bands to the park for an outdoor resistance workout. You don't need a spotter when using resistance bands.

Resistance bands are available in a variety of styles. One style includes multiple bands of varying thickness. The thicker bands provide more resistance. Most styles include an attachment that allows you to anchor the bands to a doorway or piece of furniture, as well as a strap to facilitate performing lower body exercises.

In general, the same principles of exercise used for traditional weight training are applicable to training with resistance bands. Here are some additional considerations.

Overload and Progression

As with weight training, select a variety of exercises to ensure a total-body workout. Your plan should include the number of repetitions and sets to support your goals of gaining strength, endurance, or both. Unlike training with weights, when you train with resistance bands, you will have no easily identifiable way to quantify the resistance or to measure additional resistance. As completing a set becomes easier, you can increase the resistance in several ways. You can add more bands to the handles, or you can shorten the bands by widening the base or tying them in a knot.

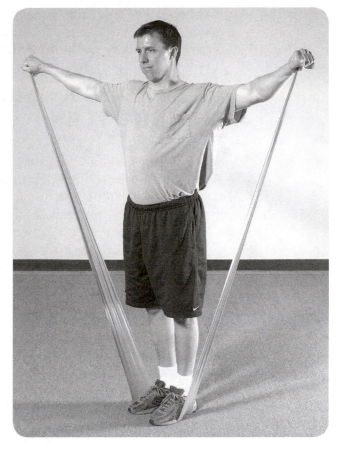

Using resistance bands helps to build muscular strength and endurance. The tension of the band (changed by increasing or decreasing the length of the band) functions as the resistance.

Regularity and Variety

Resistance bands may not provide enough training for very strong officers, but doing something is better than doing nothing. So even if you plan to do most of your training using weights or machines, resistance bands may be a supplemental tool for helping you ensure regularity. Resistance bands can also provide a change of pace from your normal routine.

PARTNER-RESISTED EXERCISES

As with resistance bands, you can replicate any exercise you can perform with free weights or machines using partner-resisted exercises. Again, the principles of exercise apply equally well, with some additional considerations.

As with using resistance bands, you will be unable to measure the resistance in pounds. Thus, you should work out with the same partner as often as possible. That way, you become familiar with each other and learn how much resistance to apply to achieve momentary muscle failure. By training with someone of similar size and strength, you can maximize each other's training effect, but this is not mandatory. Smaller officers can increase their mechanical advantage to offset their weaknesses. For example, standing on a bench or chair while a partner performs a shoulder press will provide additional resistance. Look for other tools such as a baton to facilitate performing these exercises.

DEVELOPING A CALISTHENICS TRAINING PLAN

Some officers may not be strong enough to begin a resistance training program using weights or machines. For these officers, their body weight may provide sufficient overload. Others may not have access to equipment, and in those cases, anything will be better than nothing. And every officer will at one time or another be without equipment, for example, when traveling. In these situations, consider using calisthenics as your resistance training activity.

Calisthenics training employs exercises in which one's body weight and gravity supply the resistance. Calisthenics routines work very well for developing muscular endurance, but they provide only minimal muscular strength development (unless the individual has low strength). In a calisthenics routine, three sets of exercises are usually performed, and the repetitions are gradually increased over time. Calisthenic exercises and the muscle groups they exercise are shown on the following page.

In a calisthenics training program, perform each set as a circuit. In other words, do one set of each exercise in sequence, then start again with the first exercise and proceed through the sequence for the second set, then again for the third set. To develop a calisthenics training plan, follow this sequence:

- Select exercises. Choose the exercises listed above or find ones that work on the same muscle groups.
- Determine the number of repetitions. Test yourself to see how many repetitions of each exercise you can do in 1 minute.
- Sequence the exercises. Follow the principle of moving from large muscle groups to small ones, and alternate the muscle groups. (This is done for you on the form.)
- Start the program. Do one set of repetitions of each exercise; that is, the number of repetitions done in 1 minute.
- Change at week 2. Divide the number of repetitions for each exercise in half and add a second set. Each set will have half the repetitions done in the first week.
- Change again at week 3. Add a third set of repetitions, again equal to half of the repetitions done in the first week.
- Maintain. Stay at three sets, but each week add one to two repetitions to each set of each exercise.

Use the Calisthenics Training Plan on page 92 to set up your program.

SCHEDULING EXERCISE

You can accomplish your resistance training plan in any number of ways. The key is to find an approach that works for you. Remember, this is only one part

Calisthenic Exercises

Muscle group	Calisthenic exercise	Description
Gastrocnemius	Heel raises	Hands on hips, rise up on toes as high as possible. Increase range of motion by placing toes on 2-inch board or a step.
Quadriceps	Half knee bends	Feet shoulder-width apart, back straight, hands on hips, squat until thighs are parallel with ground, and return to start.
Hamstrings	Waiter's bow	Feet hip-width apart, legs straight, arms folded across the chest; slowly bend forward at the waist until torso is parallel with the ground, and return to start.
Abdominals	Sit-ups with arms crossed*	Start on back, knees bent 90 degrees, arms crossed on chest. Sit up, touch elbows to knees, and return.
Erector spinae	Trunk lifts*	Lie on stomach, hands flat on floor, elbows bent. Raise trunk off floor.
Pectorals and deltoids	Push-ups and modified push-ups	Toes on ground, hands on ground, shoulder-width apart. Keep back straight. Lower upper body to ground and return to start. If you cannot do a push-up, place knees on ground, lower body to the ground, and push up.
Latissimus dorsi	Bent rowing (using books or other weighted objects)	Bend forward at waist, lower object in each hand until arms are outstretched, return.
Biceps	Chin-ups or biceps curls	Hang from bar with arms straight, pull up until chin is above bar, return to hanging position. If you cannot do a chin-up use a book, water container, or dumbbell and do a curl with each arm while standing. Raise the object 90 degrees and lower back down.
Triceps	Chair dips	With back to stable chair, grasp sides of chair, feet straight in front. Lower body as far as possible and push back up.

* These exercises may be contraindicated for those who have back problems.

of your overall fitness program, and we will provide some recommendations for putting it all together at the end of part II.

Depending on your schedule, you can choose to train all body parts in one session. Others may decide that breaking up the workouts into smaller portions works best. Those officers may choose to do upper body training on days 1, 3, and 5, with lower body training on days 2, 4, and 6. A variation of this approach might be to train the muscles on the front of the body together and hit the posterior muscles on the alternate days.

Calisthenics Training Plan

Exercise	1-minute reps	1/2 of 1-minute reps	Week 1 reps/one set	Week 2 reps/two sets	Week 3 reps/three sets	Week 4 reps/three sets
Half knee bends	_____	_____	_____	_____	_____	_____
Push-ups	_____	_____	_____	_____	_____	_____
Assisted leg curls	_____	_____	_____	_____	_____	_____
Bent rowing	_____	_____	_____	_____	_____	_____
Sit-ups	_____	_____	_____	_____	_____	_____
Trunk lifts	_____	_____	_____	_____	_____	_____
Heel raises	_____	_____	_____	_____	_____	_____
Chin-ups/ flexed-arm hang	_____	_____	_____	_____	_____	_____
Chair dips	_____	_____	_____	_____	_____	_____

From *Fit for Duty, Second Edition,* by Robert Hoffman and Thomas R. Collingwood, 2005, Champaign, IL: Human Kinetics.

Summary of Resistance Training Principles

The following summarizes the information you need to design your resistance training plan using the FITT acronym.

FACTOR	LOW FITNESS	AVERAGE FITNESS	HIGH FITNESS
Frequency	3 days/ week	3-4 days/ week	4-6 days/ week
Intensity for weight training = percentage of 1RM			
Endurance	40 percent	40-50 percent	40-60 percent
Strength	80 percent	80-90 percent	80-95 percent
Both	60 percent	60-70 percent	60-80 percent
Intensity for calisthenics = percentage of 1-minute repetitions	50 percent	50 percent	50 percent plus
Time weight training			
Endurance (1.5 minutes rest between sets)	15-20 reps	15-20 reps	15-20 reps
Strength (3-5 minutes rest between sets)	2-6 reps	2-6 reps	2-6 reps
Both (30-60 seconds rest between sets)	8-12 reps	8-12 reps	8-12 reps
Time calisthenics			
30-60 seconds rest between sets	50 percent of 1-minute reps working up to three sets	50 percent of 1-minute reps working up to three sets	50 percent of 1-minute reps working up to three sets
Type	Calisthenics, machines	Calisthenics, free weights, machines	Calisthenics, free weights, machines

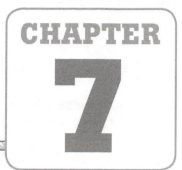

Flexibility

How many times have you felt tight when starting a physical activity? Do you remember your youth coaches telling you to "bounce it out, make it hurt" when you were warming up for a game or practice? How many times have you started a run feeling sore and told yourself that the run would work out the soreness? Do your muscles often feel stiff when you get out of your patrol car?

This chapter will teach you how to remedy these experiences. You will learn that it is not only important to stretch regularly, but to stretch correctly. You will also learn the two primary purposes of stretching: to avoid injury and to improve flexibility.

WHAT IS FLEXIBILITY?

Flexibility is the range of motion of part of the body. Generally, the more flexible you are, the better able you are to perform a given physical function.

When you stretch an area of the body, the tough connective tissue covering the muscle, as well as the muscle itself, is heated up and becomes more pliable. As a result, the muscle responds better to subsequent movement and is better prepared for more rigorous activity that may follow.

As a simple analogy, think of the muscle as a rubber band. Before you continue reading, try this experiment with a couple of rubber bands. Rapidly stretch one of them as far as you can, note how long it is, and then allow it to snap back to its original length. If it didn't break, stretch it three or four more times. Notice that it's a little easier to pull each time than it was at first. You can also stretch it farther on each subsequent pull. That's because it actually "warmed up" as you pulled on it.

Now take the other rubber band and stretch it slowly. Because it is being pulled slowly, even on the first pull it will stretch more than the one you stretched rapidly with less chance of breaking. This is how your muscles respond. Rapid, jerky movements before they are warmed up can injure them. Slow, gradual stretching produces better results.

Do I Really Need to Stretch?

Some officers have questioned the value of stretching as a warm-up. Their concerns generally follow this thought process: "If I have to get out of my patrol car to chase someone, I can't have them wait until I do some stretching." Of course not. But if you have been doing your flexibility training, you are far less likely to get injured if you have to start running cold than if you haven't been working on this component of fitness.

Law enforcement activities that require flexibility include the following:

- Vehicle dismount
- Emergency extraction
- Any activity requiring bending and reaching

Flexibility is related to injury prevention because it does the following:

- Reduces the chances of injury when suddenly going from inactivity to rapid movement
- Helps lower the incidence of low back pain

Most law enforcement officers experience back pain at some point during their careers. Some root causes for that include a sedentary lifestyle, wearing a gun belt, and sitting for long periods. Often, the soreness is the result of tight hamstrings, quads, and buttocks, as opposed to the back itself.

DESIGNING YOUR FLEXIBILITY PROGRAM

The principles of exercise also apply to flexibility training. As you learned in the last two chapters, the key questions to be answered in designing fitness programs are as follows:

- How often should I stretch?
- How hard should I stretch?
- How long should I stretch?
- What activity (stretch) should I do?

Once again, use a copy of the FITT chart on page 56 to record the answer to each of the key questions. A summary of the flexibility training tips is shown on page 108

The following principles of exercise are those most applicable to flexibility training:

- Individuality
- Overload
- Progression
- Specificity

Individuality

As you learned in chapter 3, each individual will respond differently to the same training routine. This is particularly true for flexibility. Age, gender, and previous training are contributors to these differences. The key point to remember is that stretching is not a contest, and you need to train within your limitations. For example, in a group of four people doing a simple exercise such as bending at the waist to touch their toes, you might find one who can put her palms flat on the ground, another who can touch his toes, and a third person who gets to her ankles. If you can only reach your knees, you may feel a little embarrassed. Your competitiveness may spur you to try and match the others in the group. You may start bouncing in an effort to add a few inches to your stretch, or you may bend your knees or cheat in some other way. As you will learn later in this chapter, neither solution is helpful.

The point of this example is that you have to take your individuality into account when stretching. Don't be concerned with how much farther others can stretch than you can. Although you may never become as limber as an Olympic gymnast, your flexibility will improve with regular stretching.

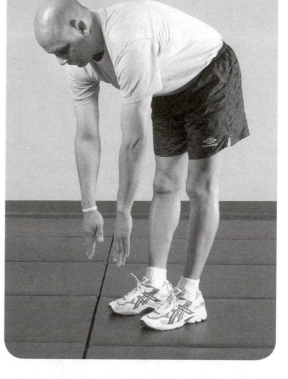

Flexibility isn't about "how low can you go?" It's about challenging your body to do more than it could.

Overload

To get a training effect, you must stretch the muscles beyond where daily activities take them. If your typical day includes getting out of bed, getting in and out of your car 10 to 20 times, walking, sitting, and then getting back into bed, you won't have to do much to exceed those demands.

Overload affects two components of FITT: intensity and time. They are defined by how hard you should stretch the muscles and how long you should hold each stretch.

Intensity

Let's try an activity that will show you how hard to stretch. While standing, bend forward at the waist and let your arms hang in front of you. You should feel the muscles in the back of your legs stretching. Hold that position for a count of 10, note how far you were able to reach, and return to the upright position. The slight pressure you felt in the back of your legs is how intense stretching should feel. You should feel slight discomfort but not pain. If it hurts, you need to back off.

Try the same stretch again, and again note how far you can reach. Before returning to the upright position, grab the backs of your legs and gently pull your head toward your legs. You will feel additional pressure and possibly even pain. That is the point where you need to back off.

Time

The length of time you hold a stretch will differ depending on the purpose of your program. When stretching as part of your warm-up and cool-down, hold each stretch for 10 to 20 seconds. Repeat each exercise three times, or until the muscle feels loose. When stretching to improve flexibility, you should hold the stretches for 30 to 60 seconds and do 5 to 10 repetitions of each.

Progression

This principle can be applied both to individual workouts and to your overall program. When you tried to touch your toes earlier, you probably came closer on your second attempt than you did on your first. If you had tried a third time, you would have stretched a little farther yet. Within each workout, as the muscle warms and becomes more pliable, you will find that you can stretch it more, up to the point of your current maximum flexibility.

Start with easier stretches and progress to the more difficult ones. For example, seated stretches are less taxing than standing ones. Over time, you will continue to improve your point of maximum flexibility. Eventually, you may reach a point where you can no longer improve without assistance. At that point, you may consider using partner-assisted stretches.

Specificity

Flexibility training is specific to the muscles being stretched. Stretching the hamstrings will do nothing for the shoulders, and vice versa. Therefore, you should concentrate your warm-up on the muscles to be used during the exercises to follow. While doing your strength training, you may want to stretch the appropriate muscles during rest periods between sets. During your cool-down, again focus on the muscles used in the preceding activity. For example, if you were doing strength training for the upper body, stretch the chest, arms, back, shoulders, and torso after the workout. Also, as you become more familiar with your body, pay extra attention to the areas that are sore and require a little more effort to get loose.

Specificity also applies to the type of stretch used. The three main types are static, ballistic, and partner-assisted.

Static Stretching

Static stretches are the preferred exercises for warming up, cooling down, and improving flexibility. Static stretching involves using body weight to slowly stretch the muscle. You should not feel any pain, and you should stretch the muscle only to the point of slight discomfort. Rather than being jerky or bouncy, the stretch should be a slow, smooth movement, and you should continue breathing normally throughout the exercise. Stretch at the beginning of an exercise session to prepare the muscles for the more rigorous activity to follow and at the end to reduce soreness.

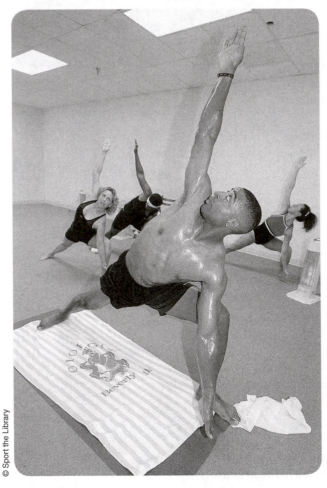

© Sport the Library

Yoga is a great way to increase overall flexibility.

Ballistic Stretching

When your youth coach told you to "bounce it out, make it hurt," you were doing ballistic stretches. Ballistic stretching involves rapid, jerky movements and shouldn't be done at full speed until the muscles have been warmed up and stretched with static stretches. You can then use them as a bridge from the warm-up to the more rigorous activity to follow. If they hurt, you probably aren't warmed up enough.

Your well-intentioned but possibly ill-informed youth coaches may have used ballistic stretches exactly opposite to the way they should have been used. If you hadn't been young and resilient, they might have done considerable damage to your body. Try to imagine what that might feel like today!

Ballistic stretches include any movement in which the muscle moves through a range of motion rapidly and then bounces back to the starting position. Many of the static stretches you will learn later can be done as ballistic stretches, if desired.

Partner-Assisted Stretching

A third type of stretching is partner-assisted stretching. These more advanced stretches involve having a partner gently help you stretch beyond a point you can reach by yourself. Be aware, though, that the potential for injury is high if your partner is unfamiliar with the technique or you fail to communicate with each other.

Regularity

As with the other components of physical fitness, regularity is essential. In other words, use it or lose it. At a minimum, you should do some stretching before and after every exercise session. As you will learn later in this chapter, these warm-up and cool-down periods help prevent injury and reduce soreness. They also help improve your flexibility. To improve your flexibility significantly, though, you should plan some additional training that concentrates solely on stretching. Even though your days are busy, you should be able to find time for stretching. For example, you might spend a minute or two stretching each time you get out of your patrol car.

Recovery

Unlike the other components of fitness, stretching does not require recovery between workouts. You can stretch every day, and in fact this is a good habit to develop. Stretching can be relaxing; you can do it anywhere, and it doesn't necessitate working up a sweat. In addition to warm-up and cool-down sessions, consider spending 30 minutes each day stretching to improve overall flexibility. You can do it in your work area periodically throughout the day or in front of the TV at night. Adding these extra sessions to your program can significantly improve your flexibility.

Balance

Your plan should include all areas of the body. These areas may vary from workout to workout, but over time your plan should include all of those listed here:

Abdominals	Groin	Pectorals
Achilles tendon	Hamstrings	Quadriceps
Ankle	Hip flexors	Shoulders
Back of knee	Lower back	Triceps
Biceps	Lower leg	Trunk
Buttocks	Neck	Upper back

When planning your warm-up, cool-down, and flexibility improvement program, select the body parts to be stretched, and choose appropriate stretches from those listed below. At a minimum, do the static stretches listed here:

Achilles tendon	Quadriceps
Biceps	Shoulders
Hamstrings	Triceps
Lower back	Trunk
Lower leg	Upper back

If you know of other stretches, use them as well.

Variety

Sample stretches for each major muscle group are outlined on pages 101-107. There are hundreds of others, and as you experiment with your flexibility program, you will discover some that may work better for you. Also consider changing your routine from time to time to avoid boredom.

Static Stretching Exercises

All of the stretches described here are important, but some are absolutely essential. See the list on page 100 for the 10 stretches that are considered essential.

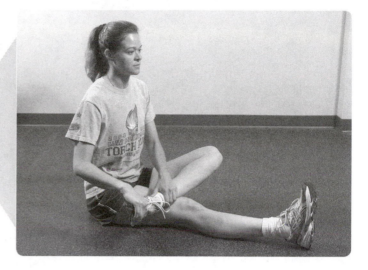

Ankle

Sit upright on the floor with one leg crossed over the opposite knee. Hold the crossed leg above the ankle with one hand and grasp the top portion of your foot with your other hand. Exhale and slowly pull the bottom of your foot toward your body. Hold and relax. Repeat for the other side.

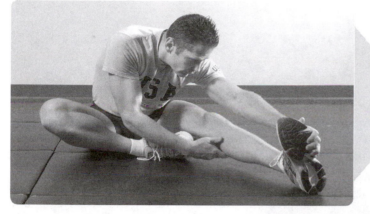

Lower Leg

Sit upright on the floor with one leg straight and the other positioned so that its heel touches the opposite thigh. Exhale, bend forward at the waist, and grasp your foot. Exhale and slowly turn your ankle inward. Hold and relax. Repeat for the other side.

Calf, Achilles Tendon, and Soleus

Stand with your hands on your hips. Move your left foot forward, keeping your right leg straight, pointing your toes forward, and keeping both heels flat on the floor. Slowly lean forward onto the bent left knee, exhale, and stretch the right calf and Achilles. Hold the stretched position. Relax, and repeat the stretch. From this position, exhale, slowly bend your right knee, shift your weight back by extending or straightening your left knee. Hold the stretched position. Relax, and repeat the stretch. Slowly recover. Repeat the sequence for the other side.

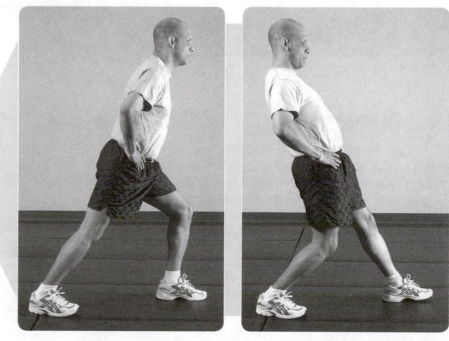

(continued)

Static Stretching Exercises *(continued)*

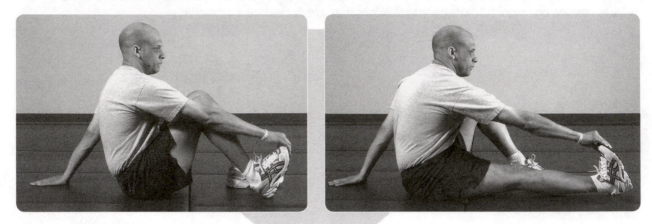

Back of Knee

Sit upright on the floor with your knees flexed and grasp the toes of one foot. Exhale and slowly extend the leg. Exhale and pull back on the foot. Hold and relax. Repeat for the other side.

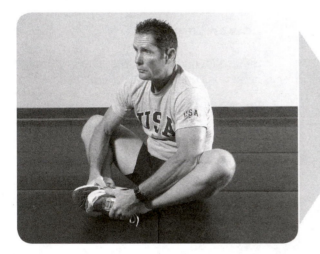

Groin

Sit upright on the floor. Bend your knees and bring the soles of your feet together. Grasp the fronts of your ankles with your hands and gently pull your feet in toward your body. Exhale, and press your elbows against the insides of your thighs, pushing them toward the ground. Hold the stretched position. Relax, and repeat the stretch. Slowly recover.

Quadriceps

Lie flat on the floor and roll onto your right side. You may support your head by bending your right arm and resting your head in the palm of your hand. Bend your left knee and grasp the front of your ankle with your left hand. Keep your thighs together and parallel, exhale, and gently pull your left heel toward your buttock. Hold the stretched position. Relax, and repeat the stretch. Slowly recover. Repeat for the other side.

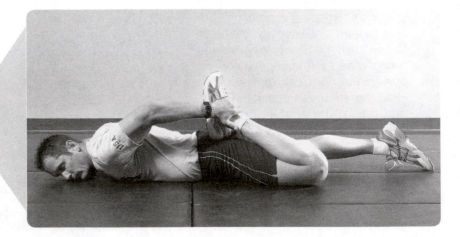

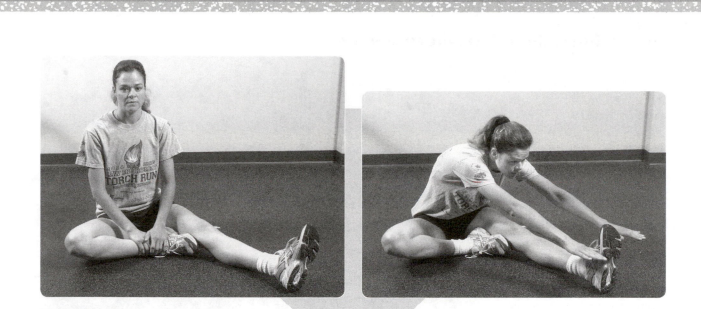

Hamstrings

Sit upright on the floor with your toes pointed up and your legs straight and slightly apart. Bend your right knee and bring the sole of your foot to the inside of your left thigh. Turn toward the left foot, exhale, and bend at the waist, reach toward your lower leg and bring your chest to your knee. Hold the stretched position. Relax, and repeat the stretch, reaching a little farther. Slowly recover. Repeat for the other side.

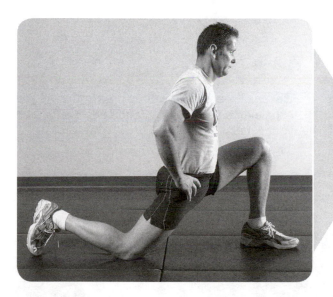

Hip Flexors

From a kneeling position, place your left foot in front of your body, foot flat and knee extended enough that the foot is in front of the knee. Exhale. Gently push the front of your right hip toward the floor. Hold the stretched position. Relax, and repeat the stretch. Slowly recover. Repeat for the other side.

Outside Hip and Buttocks

Sit on the ground with your legs straight and toes up. Place the palms of your hands flat on the floor behind you. Bend your right knee and place the outside of your right ankle just above your left knee. Slowly bend your left knee, exhale, and gently pull your left heel toward your seat. Hold the stretched position. Relax, and repeat the stretch, pulling the left heel in a little closer. Slowly recover. Repeat for the other side.

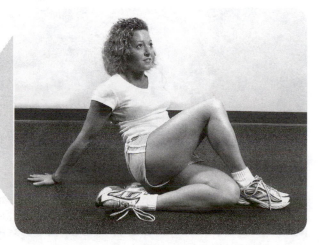

(continued)

Static Stretching Exercises *(continued)*

Abdominals

Stand with feet shoulder width apart, knees slightly bent with your hands on your hips. Exhale and slowly bend forward at the hips until your chest is facing your thighs. Inhale as you stand upright. Exhale as you push your hips forward and lean backward. Hold the stretched position. Relax, and repeat the stretch. Slowly recover.

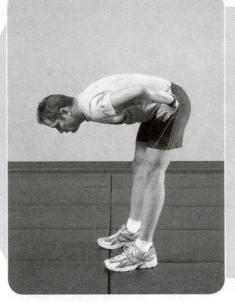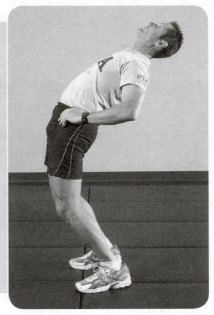

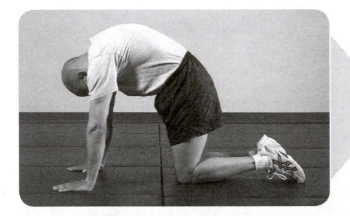

Back

Get on all fours. Take a deep breath, and as you exhale arch your back up and continue to force your exhalation. Hold. Relax. Repeat.

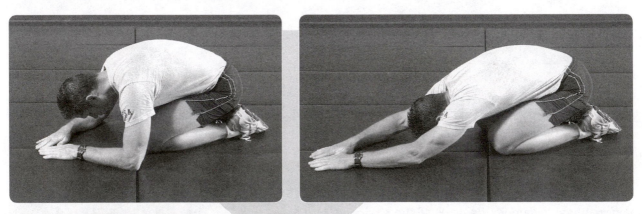

Lower and Middle Back

Get on all fours, sit back on your heels, and place the palms of your hands and your forearms flat on the ground. Keep your buttocks on your heels, exhale, and slowly reach forward by sliding your forearms and hands. Hold the stretched position. Relax, and repeat the stretch. Slowly recover.

Trunk

Stand with feet shoulder width apart, knees slightly bent, hands on hips. Twist hips to the left, and look over your left shoulder. Hold the stretched position. Relax, and repeat the stretch. Slowly recover. Repeat for the other side.

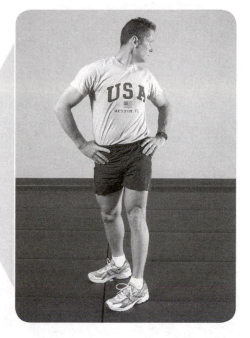

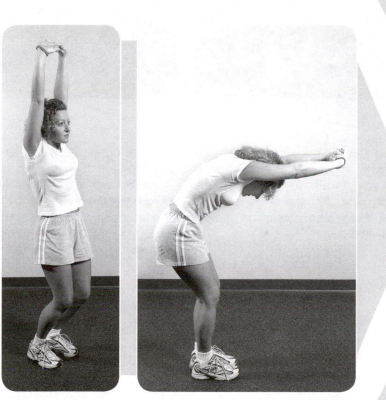

Upper Back

Stand with feet shoulder width apart, knees slightly bent. Interlock your fingers and push your palms straight over your head. Take a deep breath, and as you exhale slowly bend forward by rounding your upper back and pushing your arms to the front, palms facing forward. Hold the stretched position. Relax, and repeat the stretch. Slowly recover.

Pectorals

Stand upright facing a wall. Extend your right arm at shoulder height and place your palm against the wall. Press against the wall, exhale, and turn your left shoulder away from the wall. Hold the stretched position. Relax, and repeat the stretch. Slowly recover. Repeat for the other side.

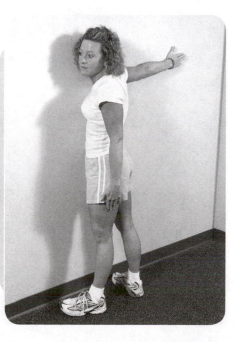

(continued)

Static Stretching Exercises *(continued)*

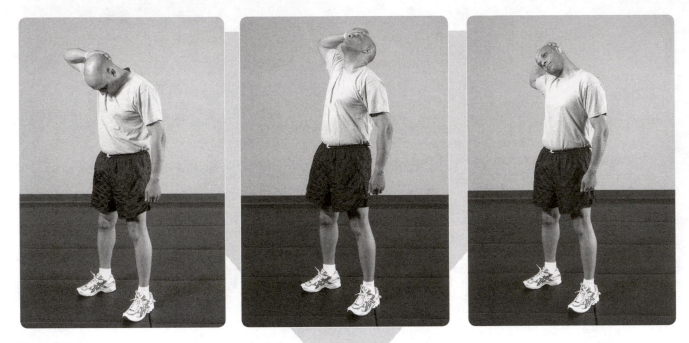

Neck

(a) Stand with feet shoulder width apart and flex the neck by touching your chin to your chest. Place one hand on the back of your head, exhale, gently press, and hold the stretched position. Relax and repeat the stretch. Slowly recover.

(b) Extend the neck by looking up as high as possible. Place one hand on your forehead, exhale, gently press, and hold the stretched position. Relax and repeat the stretch. Slowly recover.

(c) Looking straight ahead, touch your right ear to your right shoulder. Place your right hand on the left side of your head, exhale, gently press, and hold the stretched position. Relax and repeat the stretch. Slowly recover. Repeat for the other side.

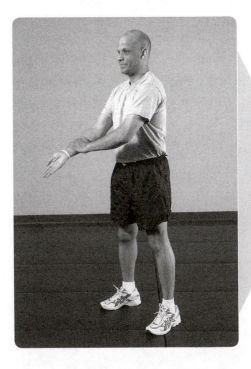

Biceps

Stand upright with feet shoulder width apart, arms hanging at your side. Turn your right palm to the front, place your left hand just below the inside of your right elbow. Exhale and simultaneously press your left hand against your right forearm while extending the right elbow. Hold the stretched position. Relax, and repeat the stretch. Slowly recover. Repeat for the other side.

Shoulder Girdle and Triceps

Stand with feet shoulder width apart, raise your right hand in the air, palm forward, and lower it behind your head. Gently grasp your right elbow with your left hand, exhale, and hold the stretch. Relax, and repeat the stretch. Slowly recover. Repeat for the other side.

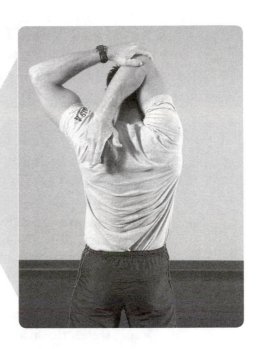

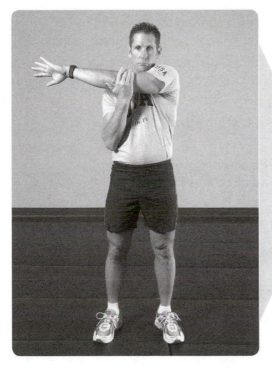

Shoulder Girdle and Upper Back

Stand with feet shoulder width apart, extend your right arm to the front, palm forward, and draw the arm across your chest. Place your left hand behind your elbow, exhale, and hold the stretched position. Relax, and repeat the stretch. Slowly recover. Repeat for the other side.

Triceps

Flex one arm, raise it overhead next to your ear, and rest the hand on your shoulder blade. Grasp the elbow with the opposite hand. Exhale, and pull your elbow behind your head. Hold and relax. Repeat for the other side.

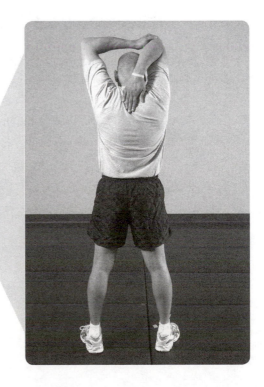

FLEXIBILITY TRAINING TIPS

To make your training safer and more effective, follow these tips:

1. The elasticity of muscles diminishes with age and inactivity. Consider these factors if you are just beginning an exercise regimen. Go slowly, and be prepared for some muscle soreness.

2. When you train, follow these guidelines:
   - Warm the muscles with some easy jogging in place or jumping jacks.
   - Start with easy exercises and progress to harder ones. For example, seated exercises are generally less stressful than standing ones and thus should be done first. It is also more convenient to do all the seated exercises while you are on the ground or floor.
   - Stretch the muscle through the full range of motion, letting your body weight do the work. For instance, when you try to touch your toes, lean forward at the waist and let gravity pull you down.

3. Don't stretch the affected area if any of the following conditions exists:
   - You've had a recent bone fracture.
   - You have sharp, acute pain with joint movement or muscle elongation.
   - You've had a recent sprain or strain.

4. It is better to do the stretch correctly, even if you can't reach as far as others can, than to cheat. In time, you'll see more improvement if you do the stretches correctly.

Summary of Flexibility Training Principles

The following summarizes the information you need to design your flexibility training plan using the FITT acronym.

Frequency	At a minimum, before and after every workout; can be done daily
Intensity	Stretch to the point of discomfort; hold for 10-20 seconds as a warm-up and 30-60 seconds to increase flexibility
Time	1-3 repetitions and 1-3 sets
Type	Static stretching

Anaerobic Fitness

Perhaps you have been participating in a cardiovascular training program for some time and routinely run distances of several miles. Yet when you run up two flights of stairs or sprint to first base in a softball game, you find yourself breathing hard. Does it seem odd that running hard for short distances has this effect when you can run for miles and maintain a more relaxed breathing pattern?

The reason is that you are using two different energy systems for the activities. As you learned in chapter 5, your cardiovascular system combines oxygen from the air you breathe with foodstuffs stored in your body to produce the energy necessary for activity. However, this energy system doesn't have time to kick in for activities requiring short, intense bursts of maximal effort. That is where the *anaerobic* system comes into play.

WHAT IS ANAEROBIC FITNESS?

Anaerobic activities are those that are done in the absence of oxygen; that is, they use energy sources that are already present in the muscle. This source of energy is limited, so anaerobic activities are of relatively short duration. For example, sprinting, pushing, pulling an object a short distance, or lifting something one time would require anaerobic energy production. Law enforcement activities that require anaerobic power include the following:

- Running up stairs
- Defensive tactics
- Lifting and carrying for short distances
- Pushing and pulling for short distances

- Jumping over ditches or other obstacles
- Running around obstacles

The most common anaerobic requirement for law enforcement officers is pursuit sprinting. Our studies over the past 10 years show that lower body explosive power and the ability to weave around obstacles while running also underlie the performance of several critical law enforcement functions. The 300-meter run, the vertical jump, and the Illinois agility test are predictive of those capabilities. Since each of these activities is anaerobic in nature, we have divided this chapter into three sections:

- Anaerobic running
- Lower body explosive power
- Agility running

Once again, you will use the principles of fitness, this time to learn how to develop your anaerobic fitness plan. The following principles of fitness are those most applicable to anaerobic training:

- Overload
- Progression
- Specificity
- Regularity
- Recovery

To complete the anaerobic training plan, take these four steps:

1. Select the activity. This could be sprinting, stair climbing, bounding, swimming, or cycling.
2. Define the work interval. The work interval includes the training distance, the training time for the distance, and the number of times the training event is performed.
3. Define the rest interval. This consists of determining the amount of time spent resting, walking, or jogging between repetitions.
4. Define the frequency. This consists of deciding how many days to train.

DESIGNING YOUR ANAEROBIC RUNNING PROGRAM

Any activity that trains the cardiovascular endurance (CVE) system is suitable for anaerobic training. Because pursuit sprinting is the most common law enforcement anaerobic task, we will use running to develop a training model.

Overload

To improve the anaerobic system, your training activities must be done at a faster pace than you would normally use for the activity. For example, if you are running, your anaerobic training should be short sprints done at a faster speed than your long runs.

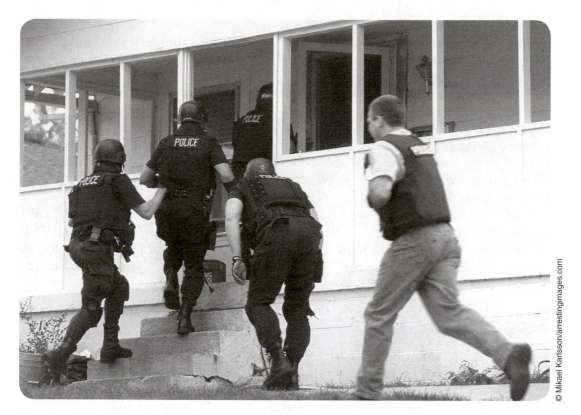

Running up stairs is a good example of on-the-job anaerobic activity.

Intensity

Because this more intense training involves a risk of injury, when you start out, your intensity should merely exceed the speed of your cardiovascular endurance workouts. This would amount to about half of your all-out sprint speed.

Time

Four variables should be considered in this part of the plan:

- The distance to cover
- How fast to cover the distance
- How many repetitions to do
- How much rest to take between each repetition

If you have access to a running track, you can use it to run known distances such as 100, 200, and 400 meters. Running known distances isn't a requirement, but it makes charting your progress easier. If you don't have a track to run on, estimate the length of a football field. Mark a starting point and a finish line. Use multiples of that distance if you decide to increase the length of your anaerobic runs.

An alternative to running a known distance is to run for a certain time. For example, you might decide to run fast for 30 seconds. To evaluate the effectiveness of your training, record how far you go during the time period. For example, you might note that in your first workout, you were able to go from the oak tree to the third telephone pole in 30 seconds. Your goal for subsequent workouts should be to cover more distance during the 30-second period.

Deciding on the speed of each repetition may require some experimentation. Taking care to avoid injury, start by running at a speed that is at least faster than your pace for longer distances. Time yourself on each repetition so that you have a gauge for planning future workouts.

The number of repetitions will depend to some extent on the distance covered. For example, if your training distance is 100 meters, you might decide to do 15 repetitions, but if you increase the distance for your repetitions to 200 or 400 meters, you could cut back the number of repetitions to 4 to 8. When starting out, plan to run a total distance of about 1 mile (e.g., 15 repetitions of 100 meters or 4 repetitions of 400 meters). As your conditioning improves, gradually increase the total distance to 2 miles.

The last consideration is the rest period between repetitions. As a general rule, the rest period should be two or three times the length of the work interval. That means if you are running 200 meters in 45 seconds, you should rest for 90 to 135 seconds between runs. The rest should consist of walking or jogging, not sitting or standing still.

Progression

Over time, gradually increase the speed of your workouts until you reach about 90 percent of your maximum heart rate. You can also increase the distance of your repetitions, increase the number of repetitions, or decrease the length of the rest period.

Here is an example of how you can put together your anaerobic running program. You can start by running 10 repetitions of 60 meters slightly faster than your regular running pace. Over the next few weeks, you can increase the number of repetitions and increase the distance and the speed. After six weeks, evaluate your condition and consider increasing the distance of your runs to 100 meters.

Specificity

To train the anaerobic system to improve its efficiency, use activities similar to those you are training for. As noted earlier, if your training includes other activities such as biking or swimming, you can use those activities for your anaerobic training. If you are primarily concerned with preparing for critical law enforcement tasks or the 300-meter run on your agency's fitness test, your best bet is to train using sprint running.

Regularity

The anaerobic system does not require as much training as the aerobic system does. As few as one training session per week will result in eventual improvements. But regularity is important. Training

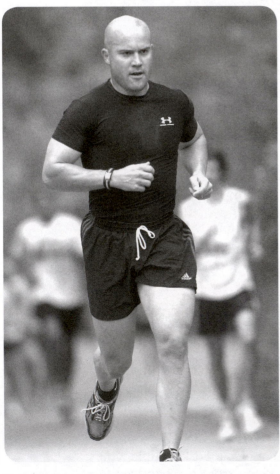

© Human Kinetics

Running (as well as biking, swimming, and sprinting) increases your anaerobic system's capacity.

less than once a week won't improve the system. Also, you will lose some of your adaptation to this type of training if it's not done regularly.

Recovery

Think back to the last time you sprinted all out or ran up stairs as fast as you could. Were your legs sore after the effort? How about the next day? Even when you are used to such activity, being sore afterward is common. The soreness is due in large part to the strain you are putting on your legs. Because this training is so hard on your body, you need a longer recovery period between exercise sessions. The potential for injury greatly outweighs the benefits of any more than two anaerobic workouts per week.

To further reduce the chances of injury, we recommend that you embed your weekly anaerobic training session into one of your CVE workouts. Let's continue to use running as an example. After your warm-up, run 7 to 8 minutes at your normal pace, then alternate faster running for a known distance, a specific time, or an unknown distance. For example, you may decide to pick up the pace for three telephone poles. You could also alternate faster and slower running each block for the next 20 blocks. When you have completed the desired number of intervals, complete the remainder of the CVE workout at your normal pace. Don't forget your cool-down.

This approach will accomplish several objectives. The first 7 to 8 minutes at the slower pace will lower your risk of injury once you start the faster intervals. Not only will the faster intervals train the anaerobic system, but the overall workout will count as a CVE training event. Finishing the workout at your CVE pace will provide cool-down from the more intense anaerobic running.

TRAINING FOR THE 300-METER RUN

In addition to improving your job performance, some of you will want to improve your time on the 300-meter run. Here is an anaerobic training program specifically designed to meet that goal. It is intended for those who have already been doing some anaerobic training. Others should train for 8 to 10 weeks before beginning this program.

Training distance = 60 to 200 meters

Training time = 125 percent of your time for an all-out effort

Time an all-out effort, then start training at 125 percent of that time. For example, if your time for an all-out effort is 20 seconds, multiply 20 by 1.25 to get your initial training time of 25 seconds.

Repetitions = 8 to 15

Rest time = 1 to 2 minutes

Frequency = one time per week

Progress to higher levels by increasing distance and repetitions and by decreasing training time, as shown in table 8.1.

A blank form you can use to develop your anaerobic training plan is shown on page 114.

TABLE 8.1   Anaerobic Training Progression

Week	Distance	Reps	Time	Rest	Frequency
1	60 meters	10	TBD*	1 minute	One time/week
2	60 meters	12	TBD	1 minute	One time/week
3	100 meters	12	TBD	2 minutes	One time/week
4	100 meters	12	TBD	1.5 minutes	One time/week
5	100 meters	15	TBD	2 minutes	One time/week
6	200 meters	8	TBD	2 minutes	One time/week
7	200 meters	10	TBD	2 minutes	One time/week
8	200 meters	12	TBD	2 minutes	One time/week

* TBD = to be determined. This is the initial time to do the distance multiplied by 1.25.

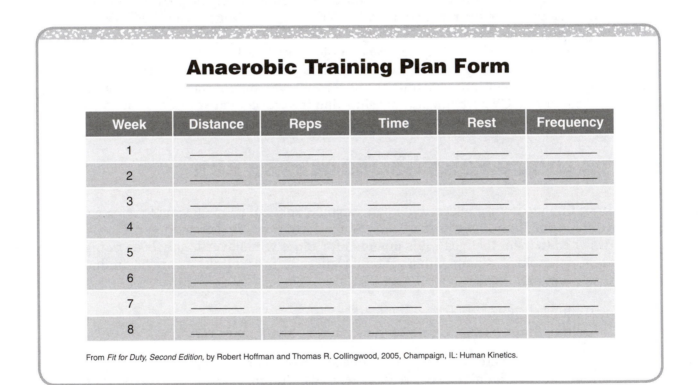

Anaerobic Training Plan Form

Week	Distance	Reps	Time	Rest	Frequency
1	_____	_____	_____	_____	_____
2	_____	_____	_____	_____	_____
3	_____	_____	_____	_____	_____
4	_____	_____	_____	_____	_____
5	_____	_____	_____	_____	_____
6	_____	_____	_____	_____	_____
7	_____	_____	_____	_____	_____
8	_____	_____	_____	_____	_____

From *Fit for Duty, Second Edition*, by Robert Hoffman and Thomas R. Collingwood, 2005, Champaign, IL: Human Kinetics.

DESIGNING YOUR LOWER BODY EXPLOSIVE POWER PROGRAM

For most of you, this will be an entirely new type of training. Those who have participated in organized sports, particularly at the collegiate level, may have done plyometric training for your sport. Plyometric training involves jumping, bounding, skipping, hopping, and lunging. Sounds like fun, doesn't it?

Because this training puts extra stress on the lower extremities, we recommend that you build a base of lower body muscular strength (chapter 6) and anaerobic training before starting your lower body explosive power program. We suggest a minimum of six weeks of training for each of those components of fitness.

Overload

When a critical task required lower body explosive power, chances are you gave close to a maximum effort. Therefore, to overload the system during training, you need to perform multiple repetitions of each exercise.

Progression

Your program should conform to this principle in two ways. First, start with the easier exercises and over time progress to the more difficult ones. Second, increase the total number of repetitions as your conditioning improves. Beginners should start with a total of 60 to 100 repetitions per training session, adding 20 repetitions every two weeks until you build up to 200 repetitions.

Specificity

A variety of law enforcement tasks require lower body explosive power, including pushing vehicles, climbing stairs, and jumping across ditches. Visualize the tasks you want to train for and choose exercises that most closely mimic the movement.

Some agencies include the vertical jump as part of a fitness assessment battery. As noted earlier, our studies have identified the vertical jump as underlying and predictive of several critical law enforcement tasks. Therefore, we have included a training program for the vertical jump at the end of this section.

Regularity

Regularity is key to all training. The main consideration for training lower body explosive power is how much time you have available. If you are already doing resistance training for your lower body three times a week, we recommend substituting a lower body explosive power training session once a week.

Recovery

Due to the intensity of this training, allow a minimum of 48 hours between training sessions. One workout of this type per week will help you develop and maintain the lower body explosive power necessary for law enforcement work.

You also need to plan for recovery between sets of each exercise. Beginners should use an 8:1 rest-to-exercise ratio. For example, if a set takes 15 seconds to complete, rest for 120 seconds before starting the next set. As your conditioning improves, gradually reduce the rest-to-exercise ratio to 5:1.

Training for the Vertical Jump

As noted, some law enforcement agencies have validated the vertical jump as a predictor of the ability to perform critical tasks requiring lower body explosive power. Here is a program we have found effective in improving the vertical jump.

Basic Program

Use the plyometric training form on page 117 to plan your training, and follow these steps. If you are new to this type of training, start with ankle hops and add one new exercise per week.

1. Warm up by jogging and stretching.
2. Perform each exercise with one set of 10 repetitions, three days a week.
3. Do the repetitions ballistically without stopping.
4. Rest for 3 minutes between each set of each exercise.
5. In week 1, do ankle hops.
6. In week 2, do single-leg hops and add prancing.
7. In week 3, do double-leg hops, skipping, and jumping rope.
8. Continue with at least three exercises per training session. You can continue with the previously mentioned exercises or add jumps and in-depth jumps.

At the completion of the program, retest yourself on the vertical jump. If you have not shown improvement, change your program by adding an additional jump, bound, or hop to the weekly routine.

Special Program

For individuals who are extremely obese, inactive, or have cardiovascular disease, we recommend that you begin with a less strenuous program. Do not start this training until you have completed the starter training program for the 1.5-mile run and are on a regular running schedule. Start with just one plyometric jump exercise and add exercises according to the schedule shown here:

Week	Number of exercises
1	One hop
2	One jump and one hop
3	One jump and one hop
4	One jump, one hop, and prancing
5	Sustain

Starter Program

In conducting our testing, we have observed individuals having great difficulty coordinating the three-part movement of the vertical jump. Those officers likely had little or no exposure to activities requiring jumping and reaching, such as basketball and volleyball. Here are some starter activities for those who are having trouble with this event.

- Skipping—just like when we were kids!
- Pogo—repeated two-legged jumping in place.
- Standing long jump—jumping forward from a starting position and landing on two feet.
- Alternate stepping and jumping.
- Stepping, jumping, and reaching overhead.

Plyometric Training Form

Use this form as both a plan and a checklist. After performing each training exercise, check off the sets, reps, rest period, and frequency.

Exercise	Set: 1	Reps: 10	Rest: 3 minutes	Frequency: three times/ week
Ankle hops—From a standing position, hop continuously in place, using only the ankles for momentum. Concentrate on extending the ankles through their full range of motion on each hop.				
Single-leg hop—Stand on one leg, jump forward, and land on the same leg. Immediately take off again and repeat 6 to 10 times.				
Double-leg hop—From a standing position, squat down and jump as far forward as possible. Land on both feet, and jump forward again. Use your arms for balance and momentum. Repeat 6 to 10 times.				
Jumping rope—From a standing position, jump up and down on both feet, landing in the same position.				
Prancing —From a standing position, push off the ground with the right leg landing forward of the body. Repeat the push off, with the left leg landing forward. Continue to alternate this movement.				
Skipping—Lift the right leg and left arm until those limbs are parallel to the ground. As they return to the ground lift the opposite limbs with the same motion.				
Jumps				
Multiple box-to-box jumps (in-depth jumps)—From a standing position, jump from the ground onto a box. Land with both feet. Step off the box, and land on both feet. Repeat the sequence. Initially, perform each jump as a separate movement. As you learn the technique, perform the movements as a continuous action.				

From *Fit for Duty, Second Edition,* by Robert Hoffman and Thomas R. Collingwood, 2005, Champaign, IL: Human Kinetics.

DESIGNING YOUR AGILITY RUNNING PROGRAM

The training principles for the development of agility are similar to those for anaerobic running. With limited time available for performing all the other exercise routines (strength, cardiovascular, anaerobic sprinting, stretching), it may make sense, from a time management perspective, to incorporate the agility training with the other anaerobic programs. Four different training strategies can be applied.

Practicing the Components of the Agility Run Test   The first step is to time yourself for an all-out effort at a distance of 30 feet with obstacles placed every 10 feet. For example, with a 30-foot training distance, you would place four obstacles (chairs, traffic cones, or anything that serves as a marker to run around in serpentine fashion) in a line, with each obstacle spaced 10 feet apart.

1. Sprint 30 feet.
2. Turn and run a serpentine course around the obstacles for 30 feet.
3. Turn and run a serpentine course back through the obstacles.
4. Turn and sprint back to the starting line.

The time to complete the course is called initial time, or IT.

The second step is to multiply the IT by 1.25 to determine an initial training time (ITT). Then follow the schedule shown here:

Number of weeks	Training distance	Number of sprint repetitions	Sprint training time	Rest time between sprints	Frequency
1, 2	120 feet	4	1.25 × IT	1 minute	One time/week
3, 4	120 feet	5	1.25 × IT minus 1-2 seconds	1 minute	One time/week
5, 6	120 feet	6	1.25 × IT minus 4-5 seconds	1 minute	One time/week
7, 8	120 feet	4	1.25 × IT divided by 2	1 minute	One time/week
9, 10	120 feet	4	1.25 × IT divided by 2 minus 2 seconds	1 minute	One time/week
Successive weeks	120 feet	4	1.25 × IT divided by 2 minus 1 second a week	1 minute	One time/week

Add an Agility Component to Your Cardiovascular Routine   Using this approach, you would do some agility drills near the end of your CVE workout. For example, you could set up sets of 10 obstacles (chairs, traffic cones, and the like) 10 feet apart in a line. You might have three sets of obstacles spaced 50 yards apart. As you approach each set of obstacles, you would sprint as fast as possible around the 10 obstacles, then jog 50 yards to the next set of obstacles. You could change direction around trees in a park, objects on the street, and the like, or merely change direction randomly.

Add an Agility Component to Your Anaerobic Routine   Adding this component would be identical to adding it to your cardiovascular routine except that you would be doing it after the last sequence of sprints.

Create a Combination Agility and Anaerobic Circuit   As mentioned in chapter 6, the term *circuit training* is sometimes applied to resistance training in which you move from one exercise to another without a rest period or perform another activity such as running between exercises. The same principles can be applied to anaerobic training by combining sprints, plyometrics, and agility drills into one routine. For this routine, you could put markers at selected points around a course for your anaerobic sprint training. Along the course, perform the change-of-direction movements, incorporate three stations where you would perform bounding, hopping, and jumping plyometrics, and then complete your

Summary of Anaerobic Training Principles

The following summarizes the information you need to design your anaerobic training plan using the FITT acronym.

Frequency	Perform the anaerobic training program no more than two days per week. One day is probably more realistic for most officers.
Intensity	Initially run at a faster-than-normal pace. Over time, increase intensity to 90 percent of your maximum heart rate. For plyometrics, start with the easier exercises and progress to the more advanced ones.
Time	Alternate sprints of 20 to 60 seconds with rest periods twice as long as the exercise time. The number of repetitions will vary depending on the length of the run. For plyometrics, start with one set of a hop, then add a jump, and in week 3 add another jump. Work up to three sets of each.
Type	Any sprint activity (running, swimming, cycling, stair climbing, bounding) could be used, but running is recommended for anaerobic sprint training. For plyometrics, use the hops, bounds, and jumps presented. For agility running, any type of activity that involves change of direction while running at speed is appropriate.

anaerobic sprint training. This way, you could get anaerobic sprint, agility, and explosive leg strength work in one routine. Here is an example:

- Sprint 20 meters, then do 10 change-of-direction sprints.
- Sprint 20 meters, then do 20 repetitions of a plyometric hop.
- Walk 30 meters, then do 10 change-of-direction sprints.
- Sprint 20 meters, then do 20 repetitions of a plyometric jump.
- Walk 30 meters, then do 10 change-of-direction sprints.
- Sprint 20 meters, then do 20 repetitions of a plyometric hop.
- Walk 30 meters, then do 10 change-of-direction sprints.
- Sprint 20 meters, then do 20 repetitions of a plyometric jump.
- Walk 30 meters, then do 10 change-of-direction sprints.

ANAEROBIC FITNESS TRAINING TIPS

These additional tips are intended to make your training safer and more effective.

1. When doing anaerobic work, you should take special precautions to avoid injury. Be sure to warm the muscles thoroughly before your workout by doing some easy jogging or running in place until a light sweat forms. Perform a minimum of two or three repetitions of the lower body stretches shown on pages 101-107 (Static Stretching Exercises).

2. Start your anaerobic running with short distances of 60 meters done at half speed and gradually increase the speed and distance over time.

3. Start your lower body explosive power training with easy exercises, then progress to more difficult ones. If the exercises feel awkward, begin with the starter program.

4. To further reduce your chances of injury, you should do your anaerobic training on days when you are rested. One or two days of anaerobic training per week is sufficient for most people.

5. Cool down after each anaerobic workout by walking and stretching.

6. Sports such as tennis, soccer, and basketball, if played with some level of skill, may be appropriate substitutes for more formal anaerobic training.

PART III

Managing the Lifestyle Components of Fitness

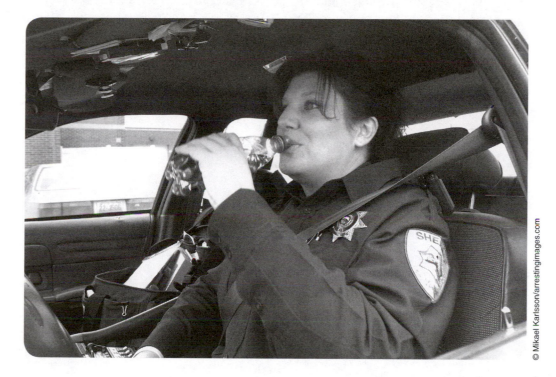

© Mikael Karlsson/arrestingimages.com

You now know about the components of physical fitness and how to develop a program to train each component for improved performance and health. But as you learned in chapter 1, there is more to being totally fit than just exercising. This part of the book concentrates on what are commonly called the lifestyle components of fitness.

The lifestyle areas covered in part III are diet and nutrition, weight management, stress management, smoking cessation, and prevention of substance abuse. Some of you may not have problems in these areas and will need to refer to this section only for general information. More likely, however, you may want help in one or more of these areas. Depending on the severity of your problem, you may need professional help beyond the scope of this book.

The purpose of part III is to give you some general information about the lifestyle components of fitness, help you understand why law enforcement officers may have problems in some of these areas, and give you some suggestions about where to go for additional help, if necessary. It is not intended to be a comprehensive treatment of these complicated subjects. The lifestyle components of fitness are the subjects of fitness training kits produced by FitForce. See the appendix for contact information.

In chapter 9, you will learn about diet and nutrition. Because this subject is a bit more objective than the other lifestyle components, it is more detailed than the other chapters in part III. Chapter 9 gives you some ideas about what to eat for improved physical performance and health. It also contains some guidelines for healthier eating.

Chapter 10 discusses weight management, a topic directly related to diet and nutrition and exercise. You will learn why it is important to maintain a correct percentage of lean body mass, again for both improved physical performance and health.

According to the American Institute of Stress, being a police officer is the second most stressful job in the nation after that of inner-city high school teacher. Chapter 11 discusses some of the stressors contributing to that status, explains how exercise can aid in managing stress, and provides suggestions about where to go for more help.

Law enforcement officers, like everyone else, sometimes react to stress by smoking and abusing substances. Chapter 12 emphasizes the health hazards associated with smoking and provide sources for additional help. Chapter 13 takes a look at substance abuse. In addition to the typical areas of concern—alcohol and drugs—it addresses the problems associated with anabolic steroid use.

Understanding Diet and Nutrition

In this chapter, you will learn about the classes of nutrients and some basic guidelines for healthy eating. You will see how healthy, balanced eating favorably affects your performance and health. Don't worry—you're not going to have to trade all the fun things to eat for seaweed and alfalfa sprouts. Rather, you'll learn to achieve balance and moderation and to develop an awareness of what each type of food you consume can do for you or to you.

Unless you never read a newspaper or magazine, turn on the television or radio, or visit the Internet, you have heard about alternative eating styles such as the Atkins diet, the South Beach diet, and other low-carbohydrate approaches to eating. Although these diets have helped people lose weight, few are able to maintain those eating routines. Further, their long-term effect on health is still being researched. You may decide one of those alternative eating styles is best for you, but we believe that the traditional "performance" diet is the best and safest approach for law enforcement officers. This chapter will use the performance diet as a basis for developing your plan for diet and nutrition.

Law enforcement officers, with their irregular schedules, may find it difficult to maintain healthy eating habits. You are often forced to eat on the run, and as a result, fast-food establishments and hot dog stands may seem to meet your needs. Even when you're educated in proper nutritional principles, it can be difficult to eat correctly. Although the information presented in this chapter will give you the nutritional education you need, a more important key to success is changing existing behaviors.

CLASSES OF NUTRIENTS

Diet refers to what is eaten, and *nutrition* refers to the value of what is eaten. Specifically, you should be concerned with the effect that food has on body function, disease, and weight control. Nutrients are categorized into six classes that encompass everything you eat or drink:

- Carbohydrate
- Vitamins
- Fat
- Minerals
- Protein
- Water

Each class plays a role in the functioning of your body and is important to your survival.

Carbohydrate

Carbohydrate includes starches, sugars, and fiber. It is the body's primary source of energy, providing four calories per gram. If carbohydrate isn't available, the body uses fat and then protein for energy. Eating sufficient amounts of carbohydrate spares protein so that they can be used for other functions such as building muscle. Carbohydrate also helps the body use fat more efficiently. In addition, the bulk we get from fiber, which is important for normal health of the intestinal tract, appears to be a factor in reducing the incidence of colon cancer and other forms of cancer and can help lower the incidence of diabetes. Some carbohydrate sources are shown below.

Sources of Carbohydrate

Grains	Grain products	Secondary sources
Wheat	Flour	Starches
Rice	Pasta	Potatoes
Corn	Breads	Dried peas
Oats	Breakfast cereals	Vegetables
		Dried beans
		Sugars
		Fruits and juices

There are two classes of carbohydrate: complex and simple. A diet high in complex carbohydrate not only provides lasting energy but also helps you cut down on the amount of fat you eat. (You'll learn more about the health risks of fat later.) Simple carbohydrate, such as sugar and white flour, digest more quickly and do not provide lasting energy sources. The recommended percentage of carbohydrate in the performance diet is 50 to 60 percent of the total daily intake. The healthiest way to achieve that goal is to increase the amount of complex-carbohydrate-rich foods in the diet, such as whole grain breads, cereals, and pasta; fruits; vegetables; and beans. At the same time, cut back on soft drinks, sweets, and desserts (the simple forms of carbohydrate), which have less nutritional value, have no fiber, and cause tooth decay.

Glycemic Index

Recent news articles about diet and nutrition have contained numerous references to the glycemic index (GI). The GI compares the effect of various types of carbohydrate on blood sugar levels and was originally developed to assist people with diabetes in choosing carbohydrate that won't raise their blood sugar too rapidly. Athletes also stand to gain from an understanding of the GI because they are interested in foods that can provide a quick energy boost during workouts and competitions. High-glycemic foods (simple carbohydrate) are digested and enter the bloodstream faster than low-glycemic foods (complex carbohydrate). Higher GI foods, which digest faster, have a smaller window of opportunity to be used for energy than lower GI foods. If not used for energy during that window of opportunity, they are more likely to be stored as fat.

Fat

Of all the nutrients, fat is the most concentrated source of calories; each gram of fat has nine calories per gram. That is more than twice the amount of energy per unit of weight than either protein or carbohydrate. But fat is not as easy for the body to use for energy as carbohydrate. Fat provides insulation for nerve endings, forms a protective cushion around vital organs, and lubricates the skin and hair. Some common sources of fat are listed below.

Sources of Fat

Bacon	Cream	Salad oils
Baked goods such as cakes and pies	Eggs	Shortening
Butter	Fatty meats	Snacks that are packaged as fast food such as chips and candies
Cheese	Margarine	
Chocolate	Mayonnaise	
Cooking oils	Nuts	Whole milk
	Pastries	

While fat is an essential nutrient, it also contains a substance called cholesterol, which poses certain health risks. Cholesterol is a naturally occurring substance in the body that is necessary for certain bodily functions. We also ingest cholesterol from certain foods. Too much cholesterol can be hazardous to the heart. Two lipoproteins (proteins that carry cholesterol through the bloodstream) play a major role in determining whether cholesterol will be harmful to your heart.

The first kind is low-density lipoprotein (LDL), which is bad for your body because it deposits cholesterol on the walls of blood vessels, blocking blood flow (see figure 9.1). The amount of LDL in your bloodstream is affected by the amount of cholesterol in your diet and is increased by smoking.

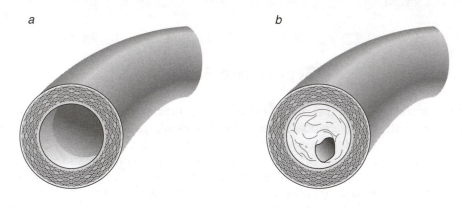

FIGURE 9.1   *(a)* Healthy arteries and *(b)* unhealthy, clogged arteries.

The second kind is high-density lipoprotein (HDL), which is good for your body. Smaller and denser than LDL, this lipoprotein carries cholesterol to the liver, where it is removed from the bloodstream. It also coats the walls of blood vessels to prevent cholesterol deposits from sticking. The amount of HDL in your bloodstream is not as much affected by dietary cholesterol as the amount of LDL is, but exercise and weight loss can increase HDL levels.

The body makes all the cholesterol it needs. Because all animal products contain some cholesterol, perhaps more than your body can use, you should limit the amount of animal products you eat. This includes the obvious (meat) and the not so obvious (egg yolks). Try to limit your intake to less than 300 milligrams of cholesterol per day. To put this in perspective, one egg has about 213 milligrams of cholesterol.

There are two types of fat: saturated and unsaturated. Saturated fat is solid at room temperature. Foods such as meat, dairy products, eggs, and coconut and palm oils contain saturated fat. Avoid these types of fat whenever possible because they raise LDL cholesterol level.

Unsaturated fat includes monounsaturated and polyunsaturated fats and are liquid at room temperature. Unsaturated fat helps lower LDL cholesterol. Monounsaturated fat is found in olive, canola, and peanut oils. Polyunsaturated fat is found in vegetable and fish oils.

In foods that contain both types of fat, such as margarine, choose products that have a ratio of at least three to one of unsaturated fat to saturated fat. This information is generally available on product labels.

Try to keep the amount of fat in your diet under 30 percent of your total daily intake. Of those calories, less than one-third should be from saturated fat. The best way to do this is to replace red and organ meats with poultry and fish. If you do eat red meat, choose leaner cuts. Cut down on eggs, oils, and saturated fat. Broil, bake, and boil foods instead of frying them.

To find out what types of fat are in your foods, become a label reader (see figure 9.2). A lot of information on food packaging may seem complicated, but you can find out almost anything you need to know from just about any label. For example, most margarine labels list total fat content as well as the ratio of saturated and unsaturated fats.

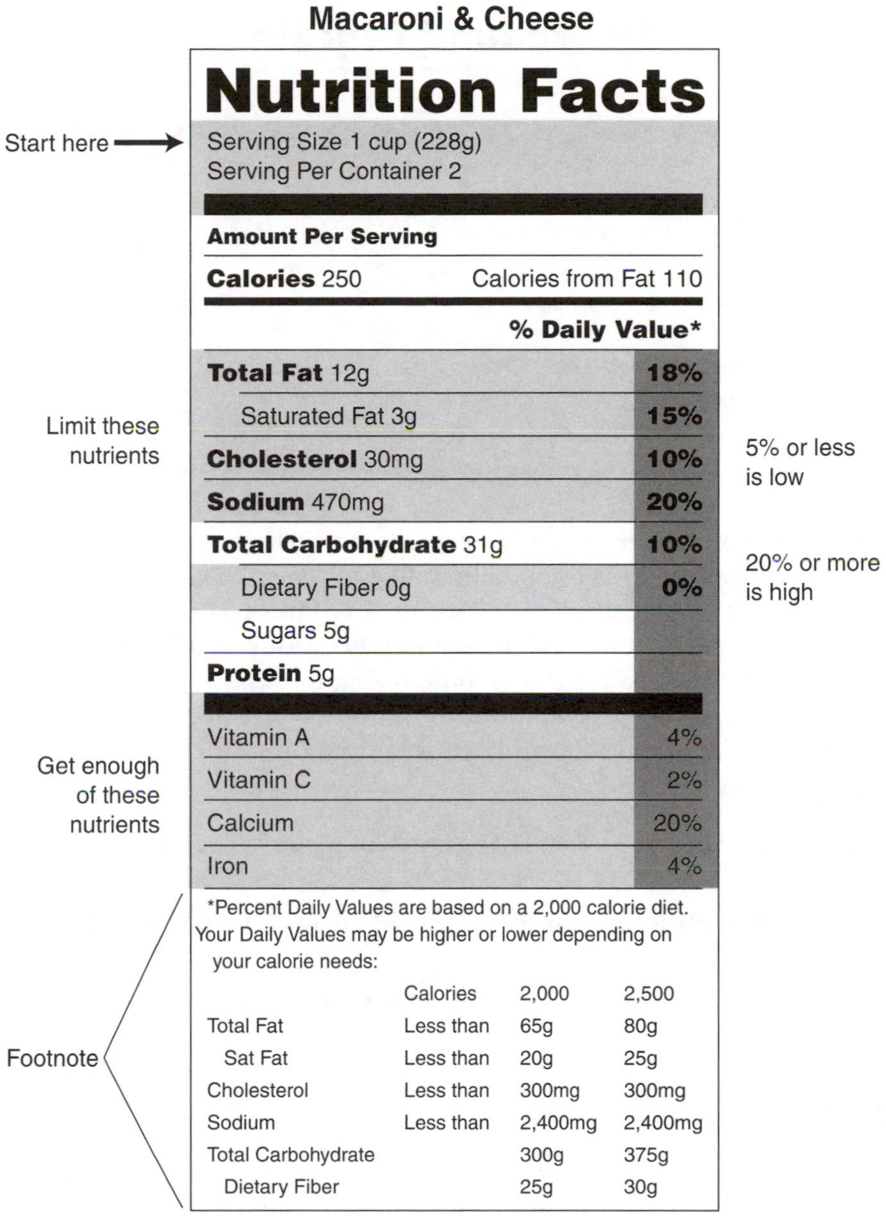

Macaroni & Cheese

Nutrition Facts

Start here →

Serving Size 1 cup (228g)
Serving Per Container 2

Amount Per Serving

Calories 250   Calories from Fat 110

% Daily Value*

Total Fat 12g	**18%**
Saturated Fat 3g	**15%**
Cholesterol 30mg	**10%**
Sodium 470mg	**20%**
Total Carbohydrate 31g	**10%**
Dietary Fiber 0g	**0%**
Sugars 5g	
Protein 5g	
Vitamin A	4%
Vitamin C	2%
Calcium	20%
Iron	4%

Limit these nutrients

5% or less is low

20% or more is high

Get enough of these nutrients

*Percent Daily Values are based on a 2,000 calorie diet. Your Daily Values may be higher or lower depending on your calorie needs:

	Calories	2,000	2,500
Total Fat	Less than	65g	80g
Sat Fat	Less than	20g	25g
Cholesterol	Less than	300mg	300mg
Sodium	Less than	2,400mg	2,400mg
Total Carbohydrate		300g	375g
Dietary Fiber		25g	30g

Footnote

FIGURE 9.2   How to read a food label.

Reprinted, by permission, from A. Jeukendrup and M. Gleeson, 2005, *Sport nutrition* (Champaign, IL: Human Kinetics), 21.

Protein

Protein is made up of amino acids, which are the body's building blocks. The body can manufacture about half of the amino acids it needs; the others must come from food sources. Protein is essential throughout life for building, maintaining, and repairing tissue. It also makes hemoglobin, which carries oxygen in the blood, and it forms antibodies to fight infection. In an emergency, when carbohydrate and fat are not present, the body will use protein for energy. Protein has about four calories per gram. Some common protein sources are listed below.

Sources of Protein

Foods of animal origin	Legumes
Meat	Soybeans
Fish	Chickpeas
Poultry	Lentils
Eggs	Beans
Milk	

The body needs a certain amount of protein every day, but that amount should not exceed 15 percent of your total daily intake of food. The healthiest way to get a sufficient amount of protein is to substitute low-fat foods such as fish, poultry, and low-fat dairy products for red meat and whole-milk products.

A common misconception is that people trying to build muscle mass and gain strength need to consume large amounts of protein. Here are some guidelines for protein consumption: First, determine your body weight in kilograms by dividing your weight in pounds by 2.2.

- For average officers, 0.8 to 1.0 grams of protein per kilogram of body weight
- For endurance athletes, 1.2 to 1.4 grams of protein per kilogram of body weight
- For strength athletes, 1.4 to 1.8 grams of protein per kilogram of body weight

Vitamins

Although the body needs only very small amounts of vitamins, they are essential for normal functioning. They assist in the release of energy from foods, promote the growth of tissue, and ensure proper functioning of the nerves and muscles. Information about vitamins is listed on the following page.

You can get all the vitamins you need in the correct quantities by eating balanced meals every day, but if you are in doubt, it's okay to take a daily vitamin supplement. Before buying an expensive name brand, compare its label with that of the generic brands. Generally, you'll find that they both contain the same amounts of the recommended daily allowance (RDA). Any brand that provides 100 percent of the RDA of the vitamins mentioned on the following page will probably meet your needs. If you get too much of a given vitamin, it may cause an imbalance in

Vitamins

Vitamin	Functions	Sources
Vitamin A	Contributes to the visual process and to the formation and maintenance of skin and mucous membranes.	Carrots, sweet potatoes, liver, butter, margarine
Vitamin B	There are eight B vitamins. The three most important are thiamin, riboflavin, and niacin. They assist in the production, metabolism, and utilization of energy.	Whole grains, nuts, milk, yogurt, fish, poultry, cheese, lean pork
Vitamin C	Helps hold cells together and strengthens cell walls. Also has a role in healing wounds and contributes to the maintenance of healthy bones and teeth.	Citrus fruits and juices, broccoli, strawberries, tomatoes, peppers, cauliflower, Brussels sprouts, cabbage, potatoes, dark-green vegetables, watermelon
Vitamin D	Aids in the growth and formation of bones and teeth. Promotes calcium absorption. Vitamin D is also produced by the action of direct sunlight on the skin.	Fortified milk, liver, tuna, eggs
Vitamin E	Protects red blood cells and aids in the metabolism of free fatty acids.	Grains, green leafy vegetables, polyunsaturated fats, vegetable oils
Vitamin K	Assists in blood clotting.	Liver, wheat bran, peas, soybean oil, potatoes

other vitamins and lead to other health problems. For example, too much vitamin A can cause night blindness and bone swelling. Excessive supplementation can be a form of substance abuse. The key in using supplements is moderation.

You may have heard the term *antioxidant cocktail.* The effect of oxidation is to produce modules called free radicals, which facilitate cancer cell development. Their development is the result of exposure to pollution, radiation, cigarette smoke, herbicides, and—cardiovascular exercise! To combat these precursors to cancer, you should eat a diet high in vitamin C, vitamin E, and beta-carotene. As insurance against the harmful effects of free radicals, you might consider a daily antioxidant cocktail. Over the years, the recommended doses have varied from 500 to 3,000 milligrams of C, 30 to 1,200 international units (IUs) of E, and 25,000 to 50,000 IUs of beta-carotene. Recent research indicates that we may not need the larger amounts. A prudent dosage would be as follows:

- Vitamin C—500 milligrams
- Vitamin E—30 IUs (New research on vitamin E suggests it may not have an antioxidant effect and that larger doses [400 IUs or more] may actually increase the risk of heart problems. A prudent approach would be to take this recommended daily allowance.)
- Beta-carotene—25,000 IUs

Minerals

Minerals are chemical elements that the body needs in small quantities. They provide strength and rigidity to certain body tissues and play a part in muscle and nerve functioning. Examples of minerals you need and their sources are listed below.

Important Minerals and Their Sources

Mineral	Functions	Sources
Calcium	Gives hardness to teeth and bones. Also involved in nerve and muscle function and the coagulation of blood.	Milk and other dairy products, sardines, dark-green vegetables, nuts
Chloride	Assists in cell functioning.	Salt, seafood, milk
Iodine	Prevents goiter.	Iodized salt and seafood
Iron	Combines with protein to form hemoglobin. Helps cells obtain energy from food.	Red meat, liver, shellfish, leafy vegetables, beans, dried fruit
Magnesium	Important for nerve function, bone growth, and muscle contraction.	Whole grains, fruit, leafy vegetables
Phosphorous	Important for formation of bones and teeth and assists in the transfer of energy.	Meats, poultry, seafood, eggs, milk, beans
Potassium	Important for heart regulation and assists in cell functioning.	Fruits
Sodium	Helps regulate blood pressure.	Salt, seafood, meats

As is true of vitamins, a balanced diet will give you your required daily allowance of minerals. Again, a daily supplement won't hurt you and is a good idea for anyone with an iron or calcium deficiency.

Calcium and Osteoporosis

One of the reasons women are more prone to osteoporosis is that as hormonal levels diminish with aging, so does the ability to absorb calcium. Calcium is essential for a strong, healthy skeletal system. Women should consider taking a calcium supplement, in addition to performing resistance training, as an insurance policy to ward off the onset of osteoporosis. Because vitamin D assists in the absorption of calcium, look for supplements that are fortified with that vitamin.

Water

Next to oxygen, water is the most important contributor to life. The body is composed of anywhere from one-half to two-thirds water. It is the mechanism for the transport of nutrients and the removal of waste products. Water regulates body temperature, aids in digestion, and sustains the health of the cells.

We obviously fulfill some of our need for water with what we drink. We also get water from the foods we eat, especially vegetables, fruits, and meats. Water is also a by-product of energy production within the body.

The thirst mechanism is imperfect, so when you are no longer thirsty, you may still not have replaced all the water you have lost. Drink six to eight 8-ounce glasses a day. A word of caution: Although all fluids contain water, some are diuretics that cause you to excrete water when you drink them. Alcohol, coffee, tea, and caffeinated soft drinks fall into this category.

You may have seen people exercising in rubber suits, thinking they are losing weight. The scale may show a loss of up to 10 pounds, but it is not fat loss. Rather, those people have lost water that is essential to their bodily functions. If you lose 2 pounds or more by sweating during a workout, replace it by drinking 1 liter of water for every 2 pounds of water loss.

BASIC NUTRITIONAL GOALS

You can't pick up a magazine or newspaper these days without seeing an article about diet and nutrition. Unfortunately, much of the information appears to conflict. One reason for this is that the articles are often based on one person's opinion or on research studies with very small sample sizes. Another reason, and perhaps the most important one, is that everyone's nutritional needs are different. Although the industry may seem to make diet and nutrition confusing, there is no mystery about what constitutes a good diet.

Nutritional goals are the basic guidelines for planning and evaluating the quality of what you eat. They are not a dietary plan per se. Using these goals will result in an eating plan that has the proper balance of nutrients (fat, carbohydrate, protein, water, vitamins, and minerals) to maintain health, minimize disease, and control weight. More specific dietary guidelines have been produced by the U.S. Department of Agriculture. They provide general recommendations for the daily servings of each food type. Rather than counting calories or grams of fat and carbohydrate, this nutritional plan assumes that if you get the recommended servings of each food group, your daily diet would likely meet the three goals of a good diet. With that in mind, we're not going to overload you with theory, but instead we'll present 14 basic nutritional guidelines. These guidelines can be used for assessing the value of any dietary plan.

1. Eat three balanced meals a day. This helps control weight. Don't skip meals, and make sure that you have the recommended number of servings from each food group. Some people find that eating smaller amounts of food more than three times a day helps them lose unneeded weight and maintain healthy weight while curbing the appetite.

2. Balance calories between the amount you eat and the amount of energy you burn. For moderately active people between the ages of 31 and 50, the

The Importance of Breakfast

Many officers routinely skip breakfast. About a third say they don't have time, another third say they aren't hungry when they first get up, and the rest say they just never developed the habit. Unstated is that many think they are saving calories as part of a weight control program. So they make it to midmorning when they just have to have a snack. Because we tend to lose our ability to discriminate between good and bad choices when we are hungry, those snacks are often high in fat and calories. That may carry the officers over until lunch, when about half hit the drive-through and the other half may have a salad, soup, and a sandwich. Many grab another snack in the afternoon to get them through until supper—when they consume 60 to 70 percent of their caloric intake for the entire day! Just in time to fuel themselves for . . . going to sleep.

Eating breakfast not only provides fuel for your morning tasks, but it also kick-starts your metabolism to burn more calories throughout the day. Consider an approach to eating known as grazing. Start with about 400 to 500 calories at breakfast. Eat a nutritious midmorning snack such as fruit or nuts. Consume another 400 to 500 calories at lunch, supplemented by another small snack in the afternoon. Supper should be about 600 to 800 calories. This approach will keep you from feeling starved during the day and help you avoid that bloated feeling associated with overeating at any one meal.

recommended caloric intake per day is 2,000 calories for women and 2,400 to 2,600 for men. Limit caloric intake to maintain ideal body weight. For a 2,000-calorie-per-day diet, eat at least 4 1/2 cups of fruits and vegetables. Eat more or less depending on calorie level.

3. Decrease consumption of saturated fat and cholesterol found in animal and dairy products. This helps prevent the development of plaque and eventual heart disease. Consume no more than 300 milligrams of cholesterol daily. Get no more than 10 percent of your calories from saturated fat. Substitute nonfat milk for whole milk. If you don't drink milk, consume nonfat or low-fat yogurt.

4. Try to consume some omega-3 fatty acids every day. Found in fish such as salmon, mackerel, and halibut, these acids provide protection against the buildup of cholesterol.

5. Avoid partially hydrogenated fat, also known as trans fatty acids (unhealthy dietary fat). This is supercharged fat that increases LDL cholesterol in the arteries. Trans fat is present in many packaged crackers, cookies, and other processed snack foods.

6. Increase consumption of fiber by eating more fruits, vegetables, bran muffins, and cereals. Fiber aids in preventing colon cancer and in controlling calories. A word of caution: Don't drastically increase the amount of fiber in your diet by eating a day's worth in one sitting or a week's worth in one day. This may result in bloating, gas, cramps, or diarrhea.

7. Increase consumption of complex carbohydrate such as whole grains, whole-wheat or spinach pasta, and lentils. These foods have good nutritional value and can aid in calorie control. At the same time, decrease consumption of simple carbohydrate such as candy.

8. Decrease consumption of sodium to lower blood pressure and aid in preventing stroke. Limit salt to about 1 level teaspoon per day. Table salt isn't the only culprit here. Be aware of hidden sources of sodium, such as ketchup, pickles, and processed foods. Read the nutrition labels on the products you buy.

9. If you consume alcohol and caffeine, do so in moderate amounts—no more than one drink per day for women and two for men. This aids in the prevention of problems of the liver and heart conductivity.

10. Eat a variety of foods that are high in nutrients and low in saturated and trans fat, cholesterol, added sugar, and salt. Follow government recommendations such as those in the *Dietary Guidelines for Americans 2005*:

    1 to 2 servings of fat, oils, and sweets

    2 to 3 servings of milk, yogurt, and cheese

    2 to 3 servings of meat, fish, poultry, or nuts

    3 to 5 servings of vegetables

    2 to 4 servings of fruit

    6 to 11 servings of whole grain breads and cereals

11. Learn to read labels. Labels list the amounts of each nutrient in a serving, but be careful to identify what the serving size is. Also understand that the ingredients (at least through the first five) are listed in order of the amount contained in the product.

12. Learn to make trade-offs. Try eating frozen yogurt instead of ice cream. Get in the habit of eating a piece of fresh fruit instead of chips for a snack. And if you just have to have something crunchy and salty from time to time, pretzels are much lower in fat than chips are.

13. Thoroughly clean hands, food contact surfaces, and fruits and vegetables. Separate raw, cooked, and ready-to-eat foods while shopping, preparing, or storing foods.

14. If you are meeting your nutritional needs while staying below your daily caloric limit, it's fine for you to have treats, such as ice cream or cookies, in moderation.

The Importance of Labels

Looking for help in a weight control class, an officer munched on a snack throughout the presentation. When the instructor started to help her develop her 500 Plan (see chapter 10), he looked at her snack and suggested a trade-off to a bag of pretzels with 100 fewer calories per serving. "Oh, no, you're wrong," she said. "I read the label. My snack has only 90 calories." Well, she read *part* of the label, missing the part that said "Servings per package: 2."

Eating well does for your body what higher-octane fuel does for your car—all else being equal, it runs better. You'll find that you have more energy, both on and off the job. If you choose to lose excess weight and are able to, you will probably see other positive changes. Your movements will become more efficient, so you'll get in and out of your car more easily and climb stairs with less effort. And you will lower your susceptibility to injury, especially to your lower back.

The evidence is overwhelming that following dietary guidelines has a direct and positive effect on health. A good diet can help reduce our chances of developing diabetes and certain cancers, ward off illness, and avoid obesity, which has been linked to numerous medical problems.

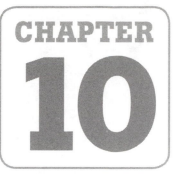
Controlling Weight

In earlier chapters, you learned that body composition and body weight are functions of both exercise and diet. For years, health and fitness professionals focused more on body weight than on body composition. According to insurance actuary tables, a person had an acceptable body weight if it fell within certain ranges for height and gender. As a result, some very strong, healthy people were considered overweight, when in fact their ratio of lean muscle mass to body fat was exceptional.

Now, although many people still tend to focus on the number they see on the bathroom scale, experts recognize that how much of your weight is fat has more bearing on performance and health. Maintaining both body weight and body composition within acceptable ranges should be the goal of any weight management program. This chapter gives you more specific information on how to set and meet weight management goals.

WHAT IS WEIGHT MANAGEMENT?

A simple way of viewing weight management is to think of the body as a system of energy input and output. Weight management is how you balance that energy.

- If the energy in the food consumed equals the energy expended in daily living and activity, body weight remains the same.
- If the energy put in exceeds the energy put out, body weight increases.
- If the energy put in is lower than the energy put out, body weight decreases.

Here is a brief description of some key concepts relating to energy balance.

- The unit of energy is the kilocalorie. A kilocalorie is technically 1,000 calories, but it is commonly referred to as a calorie.
- Food energy value can be determined and expressed as calorie deposits. Here are examples:

  1 serving of oatmeal = 108 calories

  1 egg = 79 calories

  1 serving of french fries = 220 calories
- The energy demand, or energy cost, of activity can be determined and expressed as caloric expenditure. Here are examples:

  Sitting = 90 cal/hr

  Walking = 345 cal/hr

  Running = 700 cal/hr
- One pound of fat equals 3,500 calories. For every 3,500 calories you take in above what you expend, you will put on 1 pound of weight. For every 3,500 calories you expend more than you take in, you will lose 1 pound of weight.
- Body weight itself is not the only important measurement regarding weight management. Body composition, the ratio of fat to total weight, is also important.
- Body composition is most often expressed as the percentage of fat in the body. For example, a 200-pound person whose body fat is estimated at 25 percent has approximately 50 pounds of fat.
- As you learned in chapter 3, body fat can be estimated using several methods. These include skinfold measurements, circumference measurements, underwater weighing, electrical impedance, and body mass indexing.
- Guidelines for acceptable body fat vary but generally match those defined by the American Dietetic Association and shown below.

American Dietetic Association Body Fat Guidelines

Category	Men	Women
Ideal	10-20 percent	15-25 percent
Overweight	20.1-24.9 percent	25.1-29.9 percent
Obese	>25 percent	>30 percent

Law enforcement officers should be concerned about body fat because of its effect on the following:

- Physical performance
- Health
- Appearance

Studies have shown that cardiovascular endurance and muscular strength and endurance are affected by amount of body fat. Performing the same physical task will require an overweight officer to function at a higher percentage of his maximum cardiovascular endurance and strength than a lean officer. The extra fat weight does nothing to assist performance, but it actually puts a drag on the body, making any physical task more difficult. Thus, maintaining an acceptable level of body fat positively affects physical performance.

Other evidence indicates that above a certain level, body fat (leading to obesity) increases the chances for injury and is linked to other health risks. The U.S. Public Health Service has recently recognized that obesity may be the single most serious health problem in the nation. Being obese or chronically overweight puts you at risk for cardiovascular disease as well as diabetes, stroke, and colon cancer. Excess weight is also a cause for many orthopedic conditions, especially of the knees and hips.

The U.S. Public Health Service estimates that as many as two of every three Americans is obese or overweight (USDHHS 2000). One reason for the dramatic increase in obesity has been the substitution of high-fat foods with low-fat foods. The low-fat foods that are being substituted are usually low-nutrient carbohydrate such as simple sugars that have even more calories than high-fat foods. As a consequence, Americans have been eating higher-calorie diets in attempt to control a high-fat food intake.

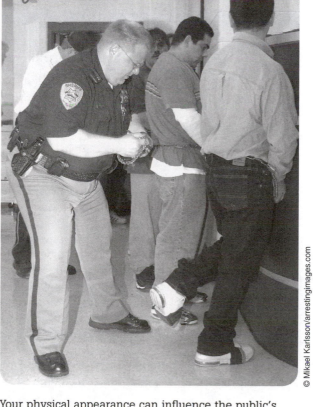

Although diet and calorie consumption tend to get the blame, they are only part of the problem. The current research on obesity indicates that lack of exercise exaggerates the effects of overeating. Over the past 60 years, there has been a significant decrease in activity levels and consequent calorie burning. Coupled with increasing food intake, this lower level of activity produces an increase in obesity rates, especially among the young. An increased reliance on automobiles, television, computers, and electronic games has changed our leisure and work habits, leading to an obesity epidemic.

The appearance issue is more subjective. Does the public have the same confidence in an overweight officer as it does in one who looks fit? Does a perpetrator think that he can "take" an overweight officer? Appearance affects how others perceive us as well as how we perceive

Your physical appearance can influence the public's trust in your ability to do your job.

ourselves. It is also a matter of pride. Most would agree that if officers take pride in their appearance, it influences how they approach the job and how they interact with others. Although appearance is not as important as performance or health, it is still a concern.

PRINCIPLES OF WEIGHT LOSS

As you know, both exercise and diet have an effect on weight loss. The evidence is overwhelming that the most effective weight loss programs involve a combination of the two. Dieting alone doesn't work. When suddenly deprived of the amount of food it is used to getting, the body reacts as it would in a starvation situation. It slows down its functions and attempts to conserve energy. Dieters typically lose lean muscle mass as well as fat, so their overall body composition remains the same. Also, dieters tend to go back to their previous eating habits after they lose weight and quickly gain it back, typically as fat.

Changing your eating habits and increasing your activity are the keys to losing weight and keeping it off. The extra calories burned during exercise, coupled with a reduction in the amount of calories consumed, result in sensible and steady weight loss. Any activity burns calories and can contribute to weight loss. Walking to the store instead of driving, using the stairs instead of the elevator, and raking leaves are examples of daily activities you can incorporate into your weight reduction plan.

As mentioned earlier, one approach to weight control is to view the body as a system of energy (calorie) input and output. A weight loss program that uses this principle is the 500 Plan. The idea behind this plan is simple. One pound of fat contains 3,500 calories; if you divide this by 7, the number of days in the week, you get 500 calories a day. This is the caloric deficit necessary for losing 1 pound a week or the caloric surplus necessary for gaining 1 pound a week. You can create a caloric deficit of 500 calories a day either by exercising to burn 500 calories (such as walking approximately 5 miles) or by reducing caloric intake by 500 calories (avoiding one Big Mac, for example). To achieve better results, combine increased activity with decreased caloric input (for example, walk 3 miles and eat 200 fewer calories). If your weight is lower than you want it to be, you should eat an additional 500 calories a day to gain 1 pound a week (1,000 to gain 2 pounds a week). For safe, effective, and realistic weight loss, do not try to lose more than 2 pounds a week. For a guide to estimating the caloric expenditure of various activities, see page 139.

Small Changes, Big Results

An officer just couldn't understand how he had gone from a body weight of 150 pounds when he graduated from the academy 20 years ago to his current weight of 270. "I eat the same things I've always eaten," he said, "although I am not as active as I was back then." If we break down this weight gain, the officer gained an average of only a half pound a month during those 20 years! That's an average intake and output differential of just 60 calories a day—less than a slice of bread or a 1-mile walk each day. The good news is that weight loss can be accomplished with similarly small changes—although we hope this officer doesn't decide to take 20 years to lose the extra weight!

DEVELOPING A WEIGHT MANAGEMENT PLAN

To control weight and fat gain, follow these steps:

1. Review your body composition and body weight. If your agency has a fitness assessment that includes an estimate of body composition, you will already know both your weight and your percentage of body fat. If not, look for a health club or health management organization that provides body composition estimation as a service. An alternative is the body mass index (BMI) you calculated in chapter 3.

2. Establish goals for weight management. Calculate your goals for body fat and body weight as part of your goal-setting process (chapter 14).

3. Identify activities for a weight management plan. Many different strategies can be used to develop a weight and fat management plan. It is best to burn or reduce calories with either exercise alone or exercise and diet changes. Exercise is more likely to lead to successful weight management because it builds muscles, which require more calories to maintain than fat, and makes muscles better able to burn fat. It helps maximize the loss of fat and minimize the loss of lean tissue. Your cardiovascular exercise plan will burn the most calories. Your resistance training (strength) program will build lean mass. Those two exercise programs will be your keys to weight management.

4. Thirty minutes of exercise per day is the minimum; exercise for 60 minutes to prevent weight gain. If you've lost weight, exercise for 60 to 90 minutes daily to maintain weight loss.

5. Implement the weight management program. Planning won't take off a single pound. At some point, you must take action. You are the only one who can make it happen. Until you have a feel for how much you eat, you might want to record your intake and count the calories. Numerous books and Internet sites are available that give the calorie counts for most foods, including fast foods.

Caloric Expenditures for Selected Activities

Activity	Cal/min
Sitting	1.5
Driving a car	2.8
House painting	3.5
Golfing	3.7-5.0
Raking	4.7
Cycling (5-15 mph)	5.0-12.0
Rowing	5.0-15.0
Weeding	5.6
Walking (3.5 mph)	5.6-7.0
Swimming (leisurely)	6.0
Bowling (while active)	7.0
Walking down stairs	7.1
Digging	8.6
Handball	10.0
Running (5 mph)	10.0
Walking up stairs	10.0-18.0

PLANNING FOR WEIGHT MANAGEMENT AND GOOD NUTRITION

The majority of this book is about maintaining a fitness program, and a variety of exercise plans have been provided to accomplish physical fitness. You have fully developed the exercise part of the weight management equation. In many respects, exercise habits are easier to change than dietary practices. Changing any behavior is difficult, but developing new eating habits seems to be the most difficult. Your lifestyle consists of habits that have been developed over time and have become automatic responses. Because eating does not require much thought or effort (as opposed to exercise), it is a habitual reaction and, as a consequence, is difficult to change.

The fact that weight management is so difficult has led to an ongoing "diet war." New diet fads are constantly appearing that promise new methods for losing weight. Any eating plan designed for weight loss, whether it's the Atkins, South Beach, Ornish, or Zone diet, is low in calories. The problem is that a given diet may sacrifice good nutrition for calorie reduction. Protein provides the same number of calories per gram as carbohydrate, but high-protein foods often have high saturated fat. A high-carbohydrate diet will decrease the amount of saturated fat but may be higher in calories that are more readily stored as fat.

Most of the fad diets that arrive on the scene are not really new but are often just variations of previous diets with a new name or promotional twist. What's interesting is that there really aren't vast differences of opinion as to what constitutes a good nutritional diet that can control weight. It's all about where to place the emphasis to devise a diet plan that is easier to follow. It's also about portion control.

As mentioned earlier, a good diet is one that (1) contains the proper balance of nutrients—water, vitamins, minerals, fat, protein, and carbohydrate; (2) helps minimize the risk of developing modern disease by controlling saturated fat, sodium, sugar, caffeine, and alcohol intake; and (3) helps maintain proper body composition (percentage of fat) by controlling calories. Chapter 9 presents several nutritional guidelines; if you follow that guidance, you will have some assurance that you will get the proper nutrition. Here are some additional guidelines to help with the weight management goal of a diet.

- Eat less "bad" carbohydrate such as sugar and white flour (the simple forms of carbohydrate). These sources of carbohydrate have high glycemic values and are low in fiber.

- Eat more "good" carbohydrate such as fruits and vegetables, legumes, whole wheat flour, and other unrefined grains (complex carbohydrate). These sources of carbohydrate have low glycemic values and are rich in fiber.

- Calories count. You consume fewer calories by eating less food. It's not about low fat versus low carbohydrate. When you restrict your intake of one nutrient, you tend to overcompensate by eating more of the other nutrients.

- Try to limit protein-rich foods to those low in saturated fat, such as fish and lean meat, poultry, and pork. These contain fewer calories.

- Choose quality over quantity. Weight management is about portion control.

The following tips may help you meet these guidelines.

- Delay, substitute, or avoid. For example, slow the pace of your eating, go for a walk instead of eating, or spend your break time away from sources of food. After you've eaten, it takes about 20 minutes for your brain to realize you are satisfied.

- Reward yourself for changing your behavior. Buy yourself a gift, do something out of the ordinary for yourself, and think positively.

- Ask your family and friends for support. Let them know that you would appreciate their encouragement and that it would help a lot if they didn't put temptations in your path.

- Consider enrolling in a weight management class or program. This can be another source of social support as well as a source of helpful information.

- Monitor yourself. Using a log will help you realize how much you eat, what situations trigger overeating, and what substitutions you can make. The Eating Checklist is a proven method you can apply.

USING AN EATING CHECKLIST

One problem with following any diet is that eating is such an automatic habit, we often don't think about what we are eating until we have had our fill. A classic example is opening a bag of potato chips while watching a football game and realizing after the first quarter that you've eaten the whole bag. Counting calories, grams of carbohydrate, or servings in a food group can be difficult. A more practical approach is to note your eating habits and behaviors before, during, and after you eat. You can use the Daily Eating Checklist on page 142 as a daily plan for meeting all nutritional objectives by giving yourself feedback on your dietary habits. Monitoring how we eat and what we eat often has the effect of naturally changing our dietary habits. Just check off each element on the checklist that you practice daily. The more checks, the better.

Although not everyone has a weight problem, almost everyone deals with the issue of weight control at one time or another. As with the other components of a total fitness program, it interrelates with each of the others. You have already seen the connections between exercise and diet and nutrition. In the next chapter, you will learn about stress. For many, weight management is one of the most stressful parts of their lives. As you will see, the positive effects of maintaining a healthy body weight can go beyond improved performance and physical health and may positively influence your mental health as well.

Daily Eating Checklist

Check off each item that you practiced today.

What I Did Before I Ate

_____ Avoided shopping for food while I was hungry

_____ Read food labels to check for saturated fat, trans fat, and hydrogenated fat

_____ Did my daily exercise

How I Ate

_____ Did not watch TV or read while eating

_____ Refused second helpings

_____ Ate smaller portions

_____ Took my time while eating

_____ Stopped eating when full

_____ Removed visible fat from meat and poultry

Foods I Added

_____ Six glasses of water

_____ Green and yellow vegetables

_____ Raw fruit

_____ At least one serving of oranges, tomatoes, or grapefruit for vitamin C

Foods I Substituted

_____ Fish and skinless chicken for red meat

_____ Broiled, baked, and boiled foods in place of fried foods

_____ Whole-grain breads and cereals for breads made from bleached flour.

_____ Low-fat dairy products (milk, ice cream) for ones high in fat

Foods I Limited

_____ Eggs

_____ Pork and red meat

_____ Sweets

_____ Alcohol

_____ Butter, cream, gravy, sauces

_____ Soda, coffee, and tea

_____ Table salt

_____ Condiments (pickles, mustard, ketchup)

Foods I Avoided

_____ Fast foods

_____ Processed food

_____ Junk food such as candy and chips

_____ Total score

From *Fit for Duty, Second Edition,* by Robert Hoffman and Thomas R. Collingwood, 2005, Champaign, IL: Human Kinetics.

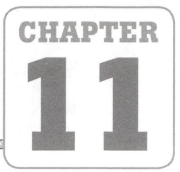

Managing Stress

Have you ever

- been driving to work when the traffic came to a standstill because of an accident?
- felt that the demands of your job were building to the point where you just couldn't take it anymore?
- had a domestic disturbance escalate to the point where you were threatened with weapons?

You have probably experienced more than one of these situations and could list lots of similar events. In addition to recognizing that there will always be some stress in your life, you need to understand that the stressors in your life can cause negative reactions. Chances are that when you were experiencing those events, you also noticed some of the following physical changes:

- Increased heart rate
- Nervousness
- Increased breathing rate
- Sweaty palms
- Headaches

- Irritability
- Indigestion
- Trouble sleeping
- Weight fluctuation
- Release of adrenaline

WHAT IS STRESS?

What you were experiencing in those and similar situations was stress. Stress can result from external conditions such as the examples listed in the introduction or from internal conditions such as being inactive for long periods. The normal stress effect or process has three stages. The first stage is when a stressor (driving in traffic, an unpleasant supervisor, a perpetrator with a weapon, or just being inactive) is perceived. The second stage is when your body reacts to that stressor. That reaction, called the stress mechanism, may include an elevation in heart rate and blood pressure, muscle tensing, increased respiration rate, and adrenal secretions. The purpose of these physiological changes is to prepare your body for the third stage—action. That action takes the form of either "fight or flight"; to deal with the stressor, we either face it head on or run away from it.

The purpose of the stress response is survival, and it is a normal reaction. It prepares your body to act, and once that action is complete, your body returns to normal. Your ability to deal with stress effectively determines how quickly that happens. Stress becomes a problem when we get to that third stage and do not or cannot react physically. One example would be a football player who warms up before a game but then doesn't get to play and is left with a lot of pent-up energy. A more pertinent example would be a law enforcement officer who is unable to resort to physical action in situations where he has to take verbal abuse. If you are continually forced to suppress physical actions, in time your body starts to feel the strain.

Stress is a natural phenomenon, and our lives would be boring without it. But stress becomes a problem when you have a job where you cannot always act physically in stressful situations. Over time, your tolerance to stress decreases and it takes less of a stressor to cause you to have the stress reaction. At the same

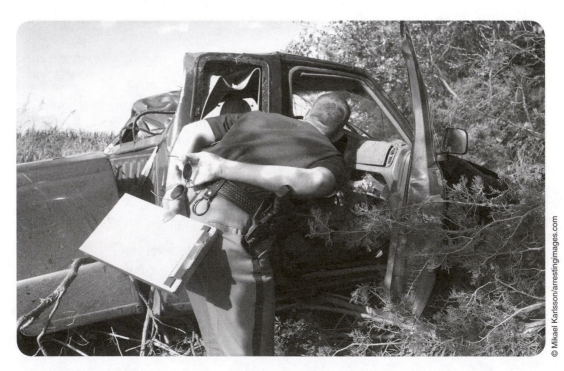

Your job can be very stressful, and you need to find ways to deal with that stress.

time, you use up your *adaptive energy,* which enables you to adjust to or deal with stressors. If the demands of your job put you in a continual state of readiness to act, decreased adaptive energy can lead to stress-related emotional and physical problems.

For many, stress seems to occur when external (outside) conditions cause physical and emotional reactions. The result is a perception that the conditions causing the stress are beyond your capacity to deal with. How well you prepare yourself to maintain your adaptive energy, how you handle stressors, and your reactions to stressful situations determine the extent to which stress will affect your performance and your health.

Job-Related Stress

In an FBI training survey of local law enforcement agencies conducted several years ago, stress management was rated the number-one in-service training need. Several studies over the years have suggested that law enforcement is significantly more stressful than other occupations, including firefighting. Indications are that, as an occupational group, law enforcement officers have higher-than-average stress-related hypertension, heart disease, digestive disorders, and low back pain. Studies have also shown higher-than-average incidences of stress-related emotional problems such as anxiety, depression, substance abuse, divorce, and suicide for law enforcement officers.

Some of the stressors associated with the job are obvious and unavoidable, such as confrontations with dangerous individuals in life-threatening situations, shift work, startle-reaction situations, and long hours away from family and friends. Other contributors include environmental work factors internal to the organization that revolve around pay, supervision, and role conflicts and the perception of an uncaring public and frustrating criminal justice system. All of these are inherent to the job.

Another job-related factor may not be as obvious. Most law enforcement positions require long hours of inactivity and boredom.

Stress and Inactivity

In the job task analyses we have performed, officers have consistently noted that they spend long hours sitting and waiting for something to happen without any physical action being required. The lack of frequent physical demands on the job contributes to the buildup of stress. Over time, the body's ability to adapt to the stress deteriorates, and it becomes difficult to find the energy and enthusiasm to participate in any physical activity outside of work. Thus, the stress due to inactivity contributes to further inactivity, which in turn causes more stress.

The research done on hypokinetic diseases (diseases due to inactivity) concludes that inactivity is both a cause and an effect of stress. The symptoms of inactivity syndrome—smoking, poor diet, and overeating—tend to cluster together and, as a consequence, lead to the health problems previously mentioned.

Adequate muscle function is needed to maintain a healthy balance within the body, a condition called homeostasis. The stress reaction is a disruption of that balance. The long-term effects of suppressing muscle activity are (1) greater-than-normal stress; (2) muscle shortening and reduction in elasticity, leading to backaches and headaches; (3) an imbalance of the adrenal glands that can affect

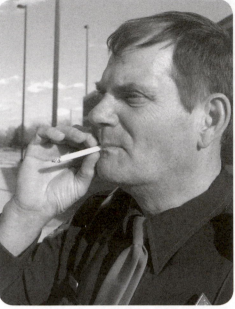

Smoking or other poor health choices are ineffective ways to deal with stress.

the gastrointestinal system; (4) heightened blood pressure and cholesterol, leading to stroke and heart disease; and (5) continued frustration at the inability to respond to stressors, leading to increased anxiety and depression.

Although other factors need to be addressed in stress management, the best way to manage stress is to maintain an exercise program. Regular physical activity can break the vicious cycle of stress–inactivity–stress.

DEALING WITH STRESS

We've seen how stress can affect our jobs and how our jobs can heighten our stress. The question is, then, how do we deal with stress? Many techniques can be employed to help reduce some stressors and avoid others.

Reducing Stress Through Exercise

Physical activity is a stressor in itself. By definition, it stresses the body. By building up adaptation to physical activity, you can increase your adaptation and resistance to other stressors. Exercise is an effective way to reduce the negative aspects of stress. Exercise can be an effective stress management tool in six primary ways:

- Exercise can serve as a release. It can release tension and anxiety and, in many respects, can substitute for the fight-or-flight mechanism.
- Exercise can be a method of relaxation. Regular exercise can be a diversion from day-to-day stress and can provide a sedative effect through natural physical movement.
- Exercise can increase energy and fatigue tolerance. A major effect of stress over time is that it uses up energy and leads to fatigue. By maintaining your energy, you heighten your tolerance for stress.
- Exercise can aid in maintaining muscle elasticity and minimize the muscle-shortening effect of inactivity.
- Exercise can increase physiological control. By following a regular exercise program, you can gain control over your body. That "tones" up the body's stress reaction (adrenal glands) by helping to normalize heart rate, blood pressure, and muscle tension.
- Exercising on a regular basis increases emotional well-being. Studies have shown that self-esteem and self-confidence are increased and that officers with high self-esteem have fewer stress-related problems. Fit individuals who exercise regularly appear more relaxed and less anxious and depressed. Active individuals report less stress in their lives. One study found that exercise was significantly more effective than tranquilizers for reducing anxiety associated with prolonged stress.

Perhaps one of the most interesting effects of exercise is that it alters the perception of stress. We have implemented fitness programs as stress management programs where the causes of stress did not change but the perception of it decreased.

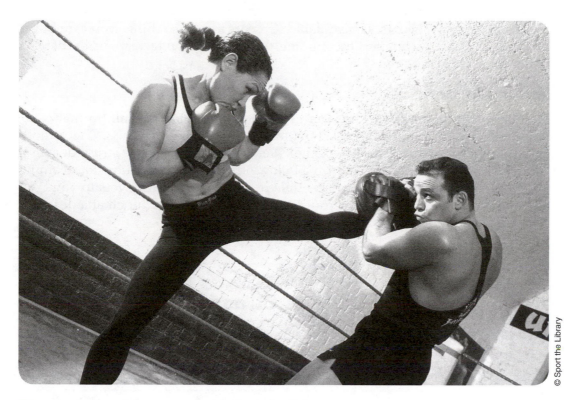

When stressed, try doing an aggressive physical activity.

Physiological Effects of Exercise

Many of you have heard terms such as *runner's high* and the *release of endorphins* used to characterize the stress management effects associated with exercise. But exercise has yet another effect on the ability to deal with stress. As noted earlier in this chapter, stress triggers noticeable physiological responses, such as increased heart and respiration rates, a rise in body temperature, and release of adrenaline. The same physiological changes occur when you exercise. You don't consciously think, "Okay, heart, beat faster. Hypothalamus, crank up the temperature a few degrees. Breathe faster, lungs. Let's get some adrenaline into the system." The sympathetic nervous system causes those reactions without any conscious thought on your part. And when the stressor has passed, the parasympathetic nervous system returns those functions to baseline. Every time you exercise, you are training the parasympathetic nervous system to do just that. Thus, regular exercisers are better able to "bring themselves back down" after dealing with stress and are better prepared for the next stressor. Officers who can't get back to normal after dealing with stress eventually break down mentally, physically, or both.

Identifying Avoidable and Unavoidable Stressors

What if exercise is not enough? Another way to manage stress is to think about the stressors in your life and plan ways to avoid them or make them less stressful. There are two basic types of stressors: avoidable and unavoidable. Avoidable stressors are those things (people, places, situations) that can be evaded or gotten away from. Examples include annoying neighbors, enclosed spaces such as elevators, or social events. Unavoidable stressors are those things you cannot get away from, such as having to commute to work or having responsibilities for children or elderly parents.

Avoidable Stressors

First, identify the negative stressors using the chart below. Think through your day-to-day activities and make a list of the ones that cause you stress. Check those stressors that are avoidable. For example, let's say that one of the stressful activities on your list is eating lunch with a fellow officer whose constant complaining about everything from his work schedule to the weather really gets to you. You can eliminate this stressor from your life by scheduling your lunch at a different time or, if possible, eating in a different place.

Avoidable Stressors

Stressor	Coping strategy
_____	_____
_____	_____
_____	_____
_____	_____
_____	_____

From *Fit for Duty, Second Edition*, by Robert Hoffman and Thomas R. Collingwood, 2005, Champaign, IL: Human Kinetics.

Unavoidable Stressors

The stressors remaining on your list are unavoidable. For each of those stressors, you need to develop a coping strategy (use the chart on page 149). You do that by acknowledging that the stressor is inevitable, then trying to find ways to minimize its effect on you. Just recognizing that there are stressors is a good first step. An example of an unavoidable stressor might be a 45-minute drive to work every day in traffic. One coping strategy would be to try a different route or take public transportation, if available. Another would be to listen to those self-improvement tapes you haven't been able to get to at home.

A key to managing stress is to accept that there will always be something that could make your life better. Being aware of the stressors and taking action to avoid or cope with them gives you some control. People who feel more in control of their lives are less likely to succumb to the ill effects of stress.

Unavoidable Stressors

Stressor	Coping strategy

From *Fit for Duty, Second Edition*, by Robert Hoffman and Thomas R. Collingwood, 2005, Champaign, IL: Human Kinetics.

Using Relaxation Techniques

Another technique to help you deal with stress is to learn and use relaxation exercises. Specific relaxation exercises can be important additions to your exercise routines. The progressive relaxation exercise below is best performed at the end of the day or at the end of an exercise session.

- Lie down in a quiet, semidark room.
- Lie on your back on the floor with your arms by your sides and your legs outstretched.
- Slowly take a few deep breaths.
- Tense your feet for 10 seconds and release. Exhale and slowly feel the tension being released.
- Tense your legs for 10 seconds, release, and exhale.
- Tense your buttocks for 10 seconds, release, and exhale.
- Tense your lower back for 10 seconds, release, and exhale.
- Tense your abdominal muscles for 10 seconds, release, and exhale.
- Tense your chest and shoulders for 10 seconds, release, and exhale.
- Tense your upper arms for 10 seconds, release, and exhale.
- Tighten your fists for 10 seconds, release, and exhale.

Although not an exercise routine per se, progressive relaxation exercises can enhance the value of your fitness program as a stress management tool.

TIPS FOR REDUCING STRESS

Following are other options to consider for reducing stress:

- Discuss your feelings with someone you trust. Try not to keep them pent up inside.
- Get away from your everyday routine whenever possible.
- Don't place unrealistic demands on yourself. Recognize your limits and strive to do your best with what you have.
- Take care of your body.

This chapter has given you a brief introduction to a very complicated subject. Delving further into it is beyond the scope of this book, but there are some excellent books on the subject that can help. Likewise, if you feel that the stress in your life is beyond your ability to cope with, seek help. Most agencies now have counselors trained to deal with the unique stressors that officers may face during their career.

The key to stress management is to control the stressors in your life and not let them control you. Starting and sticking with your exercise program is the first step. Develop a plan to get rid of stressors that are avoidable. Prepare yourself to cope with stressors that are unavoidable. Finally, learn to relax.

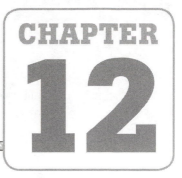

Quitting Smoking

Use of tobacco is the biggest killer in America and Canada and the largest barrier to a smoker's total fitness. Smoking results in more deaths each year than AIDS, alcohol, cocaine, heroin, homicide, suicide, motor vehicle accidents, and fires combined. Tobacco smoking is linked to heart attacks, stroke, lung and other types of cancer, emphysema, and chronic bronchitis. It also reduces the capacity to exercise because it restricts lung function and reduces the amount of oxygen that reaches the muscles and organs.

When viewed in the context of a total fitness program, tobacco use interferes with the other components. Smokers tend not to be regular exercisers. Although some smokers contend that they put on weight when they quit smoking, their apparently slim bodies can be deceptive. Smokers also tend to have poor nutritional habits. Combined with lack of exercise, their fat-to-lean ratio of body weight is often deceptively high. For many, cigarettes and alcohol constitute their stress management system. Tobacco has a negative impact on all facets of a total fitness program.

Tobacco use is one of the most powerful addictions known to humans. Despite the overwhelming evidence that it is the number-one killer in America today, 45 million Americans still smoke. And evidence suggests that law enforcement officers smoke at a greater rate than the general population.

The number of smokers includes otherwise intelligent, well-informed people who either can't or won't quit. Some continue to deny the possibility that smoking is bad for them. If you are a smoker, you may find these statistics enlightening:

- Each year, more than 400,000 Americans die from diseases related to smoking. This is the equivalent of three fully loaded 747s crashing every business day of the year. Here is a breakout of those deaths by type:

136,000 from cancer

115,000 from coronary heart disease

60,000 from chronic pulmonary disease

27,000 from stroke

60,000 from other diseases

- Sixty percent of those who try to quit smoking make it less than a year.

- Smoking accounts for $22 billion annually in medical costs and another $43 billion in lost production.

- Medicare and Medicaid alone pay out more than $4 billion annually to care for those who are ill from cigarette-related diseases.

- Smoking doubles the risk for heart disease. Coupled with hypertension or high cholesterol, the risk is four times greater. Combined with both, the risk is eight times greater.

- Some 30 percent of all cancer deaths and 90 percent of lung cancer deaths are due to smoking.

- More than 2 million people suffer from emphysema, 500,000 so severely that they cannot work or maintain a household.

- Exposure to tobacco smoke poses grave risks to babies, both before and after they are born.

- Smokers run a greater risk of premature death than do nonsmokers (see figure 12.1).

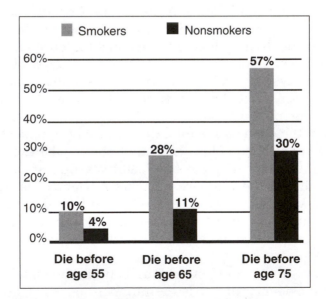

FIGURE 12.1   Premature death of smokers vs. nonsmokers.

Data from *Smoking tobacco and health*, 1989, Center for Disease Control, pg. 9.

WHAT'S SO BAD ABOUT CIGARETTES?

The harm caused by cigarettes is due to what is in the smoke and to the smoker's excessive exposure to it. A two-pack-a-day smoker spends from 3 to 4 hours a day with a cigarette in hand, mouth, or ashtray, taking about 400 puffs and inhaling up to 1,000 milligrams of tar.

Tar is the oily material left after the smoke has passed through the filter. It contains more than 4,000 chemical substances. Forty-three of them are known to cause or promote cancer and 401 others are toxic or harmful in other ways. There is no safe level of exposure for many of these substances.

Hemoglobin is the part of the blood that carries oxygen to the working muscles. One of the gases in tobacco smoke, carbon monoxide, bonds with hemoglobin to form carboxyhemoglobin. This in turn diminishes the blood's ability to carry oxygen. High enough concentrations of carbon monoxide can cause death. Smokers have levels of carboxyhemoglobin from 2 to 15 times higher than nonsmokers.

Nicotine is a highly addictive drug produced by the tobacco plant. In large doses, it is extremely poisonous. Nicotine can have different effects on the body in different situations. Sometimes it acts as a calming agent, for instance, in stressful situations. At other times, it may act as a stimulant. This may partly explain smoking patterns, as smokers meet their need for this drug in different ways. For example, the high stress of law enforcement work may make the calming effect of smoking desirable in stressful situations.

The more a person smokes, the greater the risk of smoking-related diseases. Two-pack-a-day smokers are six times more likely to die of lung cancer than are those who smoke half a pack a day. In addition to the number of cigarettes smoked, factors such as the number of puffs taken and how deeply the smoke is inhaled influence the effects of smoking.

IMPACT OF SMOKING ON PERFORMANCE

In addition to putting themselves at higher risk for cancer and heart and respiratory diseases, smokers cannot perform as well physically as nonsmokers can. Of course, there are exceptions to every rule, and you may know of a smoker who can outperform nonsmokers. But those who can do so are a very small minority.

To enhance high-level performance, the heart and lungs need a supply of oxygen-rich blood. As you have already learned, tobacco smoke contains carbon monoxide. Hemoglobin, the part of the blood that transports oxygen through the body, also carries carbon monoxide when it enters your system. In fact, hemoglobin's affinity for carbon monoxide is 240 times greater than it is for oxygen. Smoke inhalation increases airway resistance, further reducing the amount of oxygen absorbed into the blood. In addition, smoking constricts blood vessels, preventing the proper distribution of blood and oxygen to the muscles during exercise. As a result, less oxygen is delivered to the cells and to your heart and lungs. Having less oxygen means that the cells, heart, and lungs cannot perform as well.

Researchers have conducted several studies on the effects of smoking on physical fitness. Results have consistently shown those effects to be negative. Compared to nonsmokers, studies show that smokers

- subjected to the same intensity reach exhaustion sooner,
- have higher heart rates at a given level of exercise,
- obtain less benefit from physical training,
- experience disturbed sleeping patterns, and
- suffer from shortness of breath almost three times as often.

Smoking also affects bones and joints, putting smokers at risk for developing the following conditions:

- Osteoporosis
- Hip fractures
- Rheumatoid arthritis
- Low back pain
- Exercise-related injuries

It may be a chicken-and-egg type of argument, but it is well documented that smokers tend to be less active than nonsmokers. Or is it that less active people tend to smoke more? Regardless of the cause and effect, the bottom line is that smoking is harmful to your physical fitness as well as your health!

EFFECTS OF SECONDHAND SMOKE

The effects of secondhand smoke are being hotly debated. In the presence of smokers, nonsmokers absorb carbon dioxide, nicotine, and other by-products of smoke, just as smokers do. Heavy exposure may have the same impact as smoking two cigarettes a day. Besides being annoying to some, it physically affects others. Exposure to secondhand smoke can worsen the symptoms of asthma, chronic bronchitis, and allergies.

To protect the health rights of nonsmokers, smoking has become an organizational policy area. Smoking bans are increasingly being accepted as facility and employment standards. Consequently, smoking cessation is an important area for fitness lifestyle educational programming.

BENEFITS OF QUITTING

Those who quit smoking can reap many health benefits:

- They realize immediate improvements to their health, lifestyle, and outlook.
- They decrease risk to themselves and others and lessen the possibility of early death.
- Their health status is much better than that of smokers. Those who quit have fewer sick days and health complaints, report better health, and have a lower incidence of bronchitis and pneumonia.
- Male smokers who quit between ages 35 and 39 add an average of five years to their lives. Female quitters in this age group add three years.

Quitting smoking also has non-health-related benefits:

- Cigarettes are expensive and due to become more so. Ex-smokers save money.
- With the increasing number of places banning smoking, life is more convenient.

- Food tastes better, as taste buds are no longer desensitized.
- Exercise becomes easier due to improved performance of the cardiovascular system.
- Your clothes and hair won't smell like smoke. Neither will your breath, and the yellowing of your teeth caused by nicotine will be eliminated.

The effects of quitting smoking are almost instantaneous. The following outlines the immediate effects of quitting smoking.

Within 20 minutes

- Blood pressure drops to normal
- Pulse drops to normal
- The temperature of the hands and feet increase to normal

Within 8 hours

- Smoker's breath disappears
- The carbon monoxide level in the blood drops to normal
- The oxygen level in the blood increases to normal

Within 24 hours

- The chances of heart attack decrease

Within 3 days

- Breathing is easier

Within 2 to 3 months

- Circulation improves
- Walking becomes easier
- Lung function increases by up to 30 percent

Within 1 to 9 months

- Coughing, sinus congestion, fatigue, and shortness of breath decrease
- Cilia that sweep debris from the lungs grows back, increasing the ability to clean the lungs and reducing the chances of infection
- Energy increases
- The risk of cardiovascular disease is half that of a smoker

Within 2 years

- Heart attack risk drops to near normal

Within 5 years

- The lung cancer death rate for the pack-a-day smoker decreases by almost half
- Stroke risk is reduced
- The risk of mouth, throat, and esophageal cancer is half that of a smoker

Within 10 years

- The lung cancer death rate is similar to that of someone who does not smoke
- The precancerous cells are replaced

HOW TO QUIT

Quitting is hard. According to a recent Gallup poll, more than 75 percent of smokers have tried to quit smoking (Gallup 2001). Their success rates are not positive. They remained smoke-free as follows:

Less than a month	44 percent
One to three months	22 percent
More than three months	32 percent

Presenting a prescription for quitting smoking is beyond the scope of this book. For many, quitting without professional assistance is impossible. Organizations providing professional services are listed in the appendix.

If you do smoke and think you can quit by yourself, try the following steps.

1. Review your current smoking habits. Assess your level of nicotine dependence using the Fagerstrom Tolerance Test shown on page 159. As a general rule, high dependence will require professional assistance to quit. Certain things trigger, or turn on, your need for a cigarette. These can be moods, feelings, places, or things you do. Knowing your triggers helps you stay in control. Identify your triggers for smoking by placing a check next to things that tempt you to smoke.

   ___ Feeling stressed

   ___ Feeling down

   ___ Talking on the phone

   ___ Drinking liquor, wine, or beer

   ___ Watching TV

   ___ Driving a car

   ___ Finishing a meal

   ___ Playing cards

   ___ Taking a work break

   ___ Being with other smokers

   ___ Drinking coffee

   ___ Seeing someone else smoke

   ___ Cooling off after a fight

   ___ Feeling lonely

   ___ Relaxing after having sex

2. Find reasons to quit. Here are some examples:

___ I will feel healthier right away. I will have more energy and better focus. My senses of smell and taste will improve. I will have whiter teeth and fresher breath. I will cough less and breathe better.

___ I will be healthier the rest of my life. I will lower my risk for cancer, heart attack, stroke, early death, cataracts, and skin wrinkling.

___ I will make my partner, friends, family, kids, grandchildren, and coworkers proud of me.

___ I will be proud of myself. I will feel more in control of my life. I will be a better role model for others.

___ I will no longer expose others to my secondhand smoke.

___ I will have a healthier baby (if pregnant).

___ I will have more money to spend.

___ I won't have to worry about when I will get to smoke next or what to do when I'm in a smoke-free place.

___ Other: _____

3. Make a copy of your reasons for quitting, and keep it in places you normally light up. Or put a copy of the list where you keep your cigarettes, in your purse, your car, and where you watch television.

4. Establish a smoking-cessation goal. Choose a quitting goal date and a date for starting to work toward that goal. Tell your family, friends, and coworkers about the date. Ask them for their support that day and for the first few weeks. For some smokers, gradual tapering off needs to be the initial goal.

5. Prepare to quit. Use the acronym START:

   Set a quit date.

   Tell family, friends, and coworkers.

   Anticipate and plan for challenges.

   Remove cigarettes and other tobacco products from your home, car, and workplace.

   Talk to your doctor about additional help.

6. Develop a smoking-cessation plan. Many programs are marketed to aid in smoking cessation. SmokEnders, American Heart, and the "patch" are just a few. People who use the patch, for example, are twice as likely to quit smoking and stay nicotine-free (Silagy et al. 2001). Your local American Heart Association, American Lung Association, American Cancer Society, and the Public Health Agency of Canada can supply many resources, some of which are free.

7. Implement the smoking-cessation program. This involves monitoring your daily smoking count (the number of cigarettes smoked) and using various behavior control strategies such as contracting, which will be discussed in chapter 15.

8. Stick with your exercise program. Both anecdotal and research data indicate that starting and maintaining a fitness program aids in quitting.

9. Understand that slips occur. Don't be discouraged if you smoke one or two cigarettes. It's not a lost cause. When people slip, it is usually within the first three months after quitting. Here are some things to do if you slip:

- Understand that you've had a slip. You've had a *small* setback. This does not make you a smoker again.

- Don't be too hard on yourself. One slip does not make you a failure. It doesn't mean you can't quit for good.

- Don't be too easy on yourself either. If you slip up, don't say, "Well, I've blown it. I might as well smoke the rest of the pack." You need to get back on the nonsmoking track right away. Remember, your goal is no cigarettes—not even one puff.

- Feel good about all the time you went without smoking. Try to learn how to improve your coping skills.

- Find the trigger. Exactly what was it that made you smoke? Make note of that trigger and decide now how you will cope with it when it comes up again.

- Learn from your experience. What has helped you the most to keep from smoking? Make sure you resolve to do that on your next try.

- If you're on medication to help you quit, don't stop taking your medication after only one or two cigarettes. Stay with it; it will help you get back on track.

- See your doctor or another health professional. They can help motivate you to quit smoking.

10. Deal with withdrawal symptoms. Not everyone experiences withdrawal. You may have one or many of these symptoms, and they may last varying amounts of time. Following are common symptoms of smoking withdrawal:

   Feeling depressed

   Being unable to sleep

   Getting cranky, frustrated, or mad

   Feeling anxious, nervous, or restless

   Having trouble thinking clearly

   Feeling hungry or gaining weight

Adapted from American Psychiatric Association, 1994, *Diagnostic and statistical manual of mental disorders*, 4th ed. (Washington, D.C.: American Psychiatric Association).

Your body has changed since you began to smoke. Your brain has learned to crave nicotine, so certain places, people, or events can trigger a strong urge to smoke, even years after quitting. That's why you should never take a puff again, no matter how long it has been since you quit.

At first, you may not be able to do things as well as when you were smoking. Don't worry. This won't last long. Your mind and body just need to get used to being without nicotine.

After you've quit, the urge to smoke often hits at the same times and places. For many, the hardest place to resist the urge is at home, and cravings often hit when someone else is smoking nearby. As you go through the first days and weeks

Fagerstrom Tolerance Test

Check off the answer to each question.

Questions	Answers	Point score
1. How soon after you wake up do you smoke your first cigarette?	Within 30 minutes After 30 minutes	1 _____ 0 _____
2. Do you find it difficult to refrain from smoking in places where it is forbidden?	Yes No	1 _____ 0 _____
3. Which cigarette would you hate to give up the most?	The first one of the morning Any other	1 _____ 0 _____
4. How many cigarettes a day do you smoke?	15 or less 16-25 26 or more	0 _____ 1 _____ 2 _____
5. Do you smoke more frequently during the early morning than during the rest of the day?	Yes No	1 _____ 0 _____
6. Do you smoke if you are so ill that you are in bed most of the day?	Yes No	1 _____ 0 _____
7. What is the nicotine level of your usual brand of cigarettes?	0.9 milligrams or less 1.0-1.2 milligrams 1.3 milligrams or more	0 _____ 1 _____ 2 _____
8. Do you inhale?	Never Sometimes Always	0 _____ 1 _____ 2 _____
	Total	_____

Scoring for the Fagerstrom Tolerance Test

Total your points. A score of 7 or higher indicates high nicotine dependence; a score of 6 or lower indicates low to moderate nicotine dependence.

From *Fit for Duty, Second Edition,* by Robert Hoffman and Thomas R. Collingwood, 2005, Champaign, IL: Human Kinetics. Adapted from K.O. Fagerstom, 1989, "Measuring nicotine dependence: A review of the Fagerstrom Tolerance Questionnaire," *Journal of Behavioral Medicine* 12: 159-182.

without smoking, keep a positive outlook. Don't blame or punish yourself if you do have a cigarette. Don't think of smoking as an all-or-none proposition. Instead, take it one day at a time. Remember that quitting is a learning process.

What's the best advice about smoking? If you haven't started, don't. But if you have, it's never too late to gain the benefits from quitting.

Money, Money, Money!

Now that you aren't buying cigarettes, you probably have more spending money. For example, if you used to smoke one pack per day:

After	You've saved*
1 day	$5
1 week	$35
1 month	$150
1 year	$1,820
10 years	$18,200
20 years	$36,400

Think about starting a money jar if you haven't already. Put your cigarette money aside for each day you don't smoke. Soon you'll have enough money to buy yourself a reward.

* Prices are based on a 2001 average of $5.00 per pack. The cost of a pack of cigarettes may differ, depending on where you buy them.

Data from www. Smokefree.gov/guide/keep_rewarding.htm. Accessed 2/10/2005.

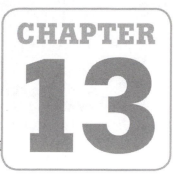

Preventing Substance Abuse

The effects of substance abuse are something you have all witnessed on the street. Whether handling a passive DUI stop or having to deal with a crazed teenager on PCP, the negative effects of substance abuse have life-or-death consequences. Those experiences sometimes make it difficult to recognize that everyone is susceptible to abusing alcohol and drugs (prescription as well as over-the-counter legal drugs), even if we use them in moderate amounts. Alcohol, caffeine, antihistamines (such as Benadryl), and painkillers (such as aspirin and ibuprofen) are legal substances that many of us use on a regular basis. If taken in excessive amounts, all can have serious physical, emotional, and social consequences. Substance abuse can destroy careers, families, and the individuals themselves. As an officer, you are concerned with this issue from several perspectives:

- Your own well-being
- The well-being of your family
- The public you serve
- The model you project
- The law you are sworn to uphold

The implications of substance abuse come into play in three main areas: legal, social, and health. You are abundantly familiar with the legal implications. The societal implications can only be discussed in general terms because an in-depth discussion is beyond the scope of this book. Therefore, this section will concentrate on the health and performance effects of the three substances most likely to be abused by you and your family: alcohol, drugs (both recreational and prescription), and performance-enhancing drugs such as steroids (technically a drug, but used for a different purpose than we commonly think of when we refer to the "drug problem").

ALCOHOL

Alcohol abuse affects many lives. As with all drugs, there are legal, social, and health consequences associated with its misuse. Although alcohol use itself is legal, every day thousands of people break the law by getting behind the wheel of a vehicle when their blood-alcohol content is above the legal limit. Although few people who do this equate it with a burglary or other crime, it is no less illegal, and the potential consequences are horrible to consider. Half of all motor vehicle accidents in the United States involve alcohol. Every day, innocent men, women, and children are struck down before their time by drunk drivers. The public outrage has grown to the point where laws are becoming stricter. The amount of alcohol in the blood required to declare someone under the influence gets lower with the passage of increasingly tougher legislation.

Other problems are associated with the abuse of alcohol. Many families are destroyed because of the destructive use of alcohol by one or more members. By some definitions, use of alcohol in any quantity is a problem if it affects family life. A common problem behavior stemming from drinking is domestic violence. How many calls have you answered for this problem? And as you well know, the scenario may involve anything from disturbing the neighbors to spousal abuse.

Problems with drinking often carry over to the job and manifest themselves in different ways. Drinkers are late for work more often and over time usually develop attendance problems. Their performance on the job deteriorates as they deal with drowsiness, headaches, lack of concentration, and other symptoms of hangovers. Their appearance may be affected, and being around them may become offensive to the senses of their fellow employees.

According to the National Institute on Alcohol Abuse and Alcoholism, about 7 percent of adults can be categorized as alcohol abusers or as alcohol dependent. Alcohol consumption increases with income and is more prevalent among males than among females. Alcoholism appears to have a genetic component;

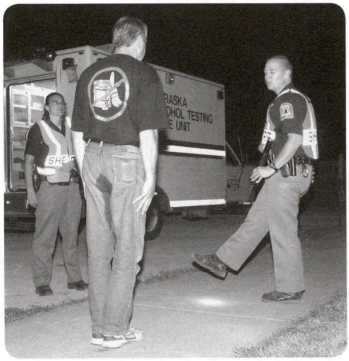

© Mikael Karlsson/arrestingimages.com

Alcohol greatly affects your job, whether it's dealing with DUIs or your own use of alcohol.

that is, the offspring of alcoholics are at high risk for becoming alcoholics themselves.

Alcohol is often available in social settings, and there is nothing wrong with being a social drinker. Unfortunately, many people have forgotten how to drink socially. Here are a few tips on drinking socially.

- Never accept a drink unless you want one.
- Know your limit.
- Eat while you drink.
- Sip your drinks; don't gulp them.
- Alternate alcoholic and nonalcoholic beverages.
- Don't drink to relax.
- Don't drink to forget your problems.
- Don't drink and drive.

Finally, there is the health issue. Although generally considered to be underreported, alcohol-related illnesses are still responsible for 4 percent of deaths worldwide (Room et al. 2005). Certain cancers, liver damage, impotency, and other nerve disorders have all been connected with alcohol abuse. It also causes digestive abnormalities that can result in nutritional deficiencies. In addition, alcohol blocks the ability of the blood to carry oxygen to the working muscles by attaching to hemoglobin, the oxygen-carrying element of the blood. This detracts from performance in all activities requiring cardiovascular endurance.

Generally, people with drinking problems need professional help to quit. The all-important first step is recognition of the problem. The tendency is to deny that a problem exists and to claim that you can stop at any time. Any number of tools are available for assessing whether or not alcohol is a problem in your life. One such tool is the CAGE Alcohol Abuse Checklist below.

CAGE Alcohol Abuse Checklist

Answer yes or no to the following four questions.

1. Have you ever felt you should cut down on your drinking? _____
2. Have people annoyed you by criticizing your drinking? _____
3. Have you ever felt bad or guilty about your drinking?_____
4. Have you ever had a drink first thing in the morning to steady your nerves or get rid of a hangover?_____

If you answered yes to any of the questions, you may be abusing alcohol and should consider the need for professional guidance.

From *Fit for Duty, Second Edition,* by Robert Hoffman and Thomas R. Collingwood, 2005, Champaign, IL: Human Kinetics. Adapted from J. Ewing, 1984, "The CAGE Questionnaire," *Journal of the American Medical Association* 252: 1905-1907.

DRUGS

We all know that the use of street drugs (or recreational drugs) is against the law. We've also been exposed to enough information that we know the harm street drugs can do to our health. We read in the paper every day about someone dying from an overdose. The statistics relating crime to drug use are staggering. Yet people continue to use and abuse drugs. Why? Because they are so powerfully addictive that the only sure way to stay off drugs is never to get on them to begin with.

As with alcohol, treatment is best left to the professionals. Recognizing a problem with either yourself or someone you care about is the critical first step. The more difficult step is doing something about it.

Although far more attention is concentrated on illegal drugs, the abuse of prescription drugs is no less harmful. They can have the same debilitating effects on health, performance, and relationships as do street drugs. In some ways, they may have more potential for danger, because often the abusers are otherwise law-abiding people who may never be suspected of having a problem and may not realize it themselves.

There is growing concern about the abuse of over-the-counter drugs. Anti-inflammatories, if taken in excess, can cause serious gastrointestinal conditions. Overuse of antihistamines can cause mental attention and alertness difficulties. Caffeine, whether taken in tablet form or through excessive use of coffee, tea, and cola drinks, can cause heart arrhythmias. Although not in the same category as alcohol, in terms of negative effects, we must be alert to the abuse of controlled and prescription drugs as well.

We will assume that drug abuse is not a problem for the readers of this book, but that it may be for people they care about. Some signs that a person is having a problem with drugs include the following behavioral changes:

- Keeping odd hours
- Otherwise unexplained loss of weight
- Personality change—becoming withdrawn
- Loss of interest in school, work, and other activities
- Deterioration of appearance

Numerous counseling services are available for those with drug abuse problems. The hardest part is getting those who have a problem to admit they need help. Having someone who cares makes it much easier to face up to the problem and try to do something about it. Although dealing with a drug abuse problem can be a very trying time for all concerned, the following tips may help you cope with the situation a little bit better:

- Don't try to deal with someone under the influence.
- Don't cover up or make excuses for the person.
- Don't make an issue of seeking treatment.
- Provide a supportive home environment.
- Don't expect overnight changes.

PERFORMANCE-ENHANCING DRUGS AND STEROIDS

Everyone nowadays is looking to gain an "edge." Performance-enhancing drugs have been around for decades, but they were used predominantly by high-level athletes. That has all changed. Today, many have the attitude that use of steroids is not just okay, but necessary. An example of that attitude is some SWAT team members we trained who were advocates of steroid use to keep a step ahead of the "bad guys." This trend is seen in surveys where steroid use has been documented among American males as young as junior high school age. Steroid use is also growing among American females.

Many athletes use steroids to enhance athletic performance (the latest scandal in baseball highlights the severity of the problem), but the desire to increase muscle mass for appearance is equally strong. A serious misperception is that using performance-enhancing drugs can be a shortcut to muscle and fitness gains—that you can get the same effect without having to train hard. This phenomenon does not just apply to steroids but to other substances such as creatine. Whereas there are data to show the negative effects of steroids, very little data are available on the safety of other performance-enhancing drugs. One thing we can be sure of is that new performance-enhancing drugs will be developed in the future.

Experts are also raising questions about excessive use of vitamin and mineral supplements. If the daily intake of vitamins and minerals greatly exceeds the recommended daily allowance, negative side effects can result. In addition, taking certain vitamins and minerals in excess can block other vitamins and minerals from performing their roles in healthy body functioning.

Still, the major performance-enhancing drug abuse is that of steroids. Steroid use can result in severe physical as well as psychological changes. These include increased cholesterol, triglycerides, and glucose; shrunken testicles; irritability; and "roid rage." Steroid use increases the risk of liver cancer, hepatitis, hypertension, and diabetes. Despite how well publicized these destructive results of using steroids are, many users are unable to think of anything other than the short-term gains in strength and size.

Symptoms of steroid use include the following:

- Mood swings and increased aggressiveness
- Acne
- Voice lowering (in females)
- Increases in facial and body hair
- Above-normal gains in muscle mass

Steroid use is becoming a serious problem within law enforcement. Recently, four Oklahoma police officers were terminated for using steroids. The excuse given by the officers was that the steroids were needed to prepare themselves physically for use-of-force situations and to have the confidence to do the job. This negative motivation is not only unprofessional, irresponsible, and unethical, but unnecessary. Although the officers' concern is legitimate, the fitness program outlined is this book would have prepared them physically and given them the confidence they needed to perform their job tasks.

Unfortunately, steroids offer the age-old promise of being able to reach a goal without having to do the hard work necessary to get there. The issue when considering the use of any performance-enhancement drug or supplement is to ask yourself, "Can I get the same effect by having a quality training and dietary program—without the dangerous side effects?"

This chapter only scratches the surface of the issues surrounding substance abuse. The intent was to increase awareness of the problem and reinforce the need to seek professional help. The hope is that you will never need the information provided in this chapter, but unfortunately, that is probably not realistic. If you do suspect a problem, taking some action is better than sitting back and letting the problem get worse, whether it's yours or someone else's.

As with stress management, one of the best things you can do to avoid the lure of any substance is to follow your exercise program. Surveys of individuals who abuse alcohol and drugs suggest that they do it because it makes them feel good, it allows them to relax, it gives them an escape from the pressures and stresses of life, and that it is an uncontrollable habit. Those same answers are found in surveys of why habitual exercisers continue in their fitness program.

At any time, you can look at your health habits and ask the question: "Am I on a health-enhancing or health-compromising lifestyle path?" Healthy behaviors tend to cluster together, and vice versa. We have seen many instances where individuals who were abusing drugs stopped after involvement with an exercise program. Although sustaining an exercise program is just one behavior, it is one with which unhealthy choices don't fit very well. Over time, the fitness lifestyle can support the prevention of substance abuse.

Maintaining Your Fitness

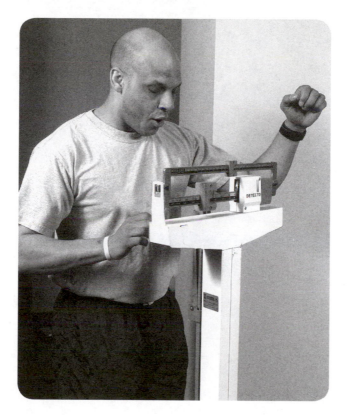

You now have all the information you need to get started on a fitness program to improve your health and performance. Part I helped you determine your current level of physical fitness and gave you a starting point to build from. Part II gave you the information you need to design a program to improve your cardiovascular endurance, muscular strength and endurance, flexibility, and anaerobic power. In part III, you learned some basic information about the life-style components of fitness.

Part IV ties all the previous information together. You were exposed to some elements of goal setting in chapters 4 through 7. Chapter 14 presents a more formal approach to this key subject. You will learn why it is important to set goals, both for fitness and in other areas of your life. We present an acronym we call CHAMPS to help you follow the goal-setting procedure as you learn the principles. Forms are included that will facilitate your own goal-setting process.

Even the most dedicated, experienced exercisers have days when they find it hard to get started. People also fall off their programs occasionally for reasons beyond their control, such as injuries. Chapter 15 describes some potential pitfalls and sidetracks to watch for in your ongoing fitness efforts, as well as some motivational tools to use at those times when you may need a boost. You will also learn about fitness contracts and how they may help you adhere to your program.

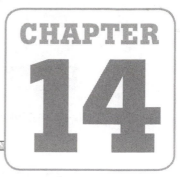

Setting Fitness Goals

In chapter 3, you learned about fitness assessments. In part II, you learned how to train using the components of physical fitness. Part III gave you some information about the lifestyle components of fitness. Throughout those chapters, you gained some insights into what kind of goals you might consider for your own program. The purpose of this chapter is to give you some more specific information about the process of goal setting. You'll be focusing on fitness goals to define the expectations for maintaining and improving fitness, but goal setting can help you in all areas of your life, not just your fitness program.

Most of us perform better when we have a specific goal to work toward. A goal gives meaning to our actions, helps establish intermediate benchmarks for checking progress, and provides motivation. Studies have shown that people adhere to programs better when they set goals and that the adherence is even stronger when they write down their goals.

Goal setting should be an ongoing, systematic, and progressive process. As you learn more about your abilities, you may want to update your goals to make them more realistic. And as you attain a goal, set a new challenge for yourself. Your expectations should just exceed your reach!

If you are beginning a fitness program, your approach to goal setting may be different than that of more experienced exercisers. The latter probably maintain a habit of regular exercise and have a clearer idea of their physical performance capabilities. The CHAMPS goal-setting approach (see a detailed explanation on pages 171-173) is geared especially toward the beginner, but more experienced exercisers will find the approach helpful as well.

DETERMINING YOUR FITNESS GOALS

To develop goals, you must know where you are now, have some idea of where you want to go, consider what it's going to take to get there, and have a way to evaluate your progress. Here are four steps to help you visualize this process.

Step 1: Know Where You Are Now   You can evaluate your present condition in several ways. One would be the assessments you did in chapter 3. Another might be the results of a doctor's examination. Yet a third could be your own self-analysis. Obviously, the first two are more objective, but all are effective if they give you a clear idea of where you are starting from.

Step 2: Know Where You Want to Go   Your goal will usually be based on a need or a desire. For example, your department or agency may have standards that you failed to meet on your assessment. Your doctor may tell you that you need to make lifestyle changes to avoid serious health problems. Or you may decide that you just want to look better.

Attaining any of these results may be your long-term goal, but it may take a while to get there. To avoid discouragement, you should set short-term goals. For example, you might set a goal of 10 percent improvement in fitness every eight weeks until you reach the agency standard.

Make sure the goals you set are challenging yet attainable. If you were deficient on the 12-minute run, for example, planning to win next year's Boston Marathon is probably not a reasonable goal. In fact, if you are not sure how high to set your intermediate goals, it is probably better to set them a little too low than a little too high. Although your goals should be challenging, reaching the low goal will probably be a more positive experience than failing on the high one. You can always readjust.

For many, performance goals are more effective than outcome goals. For example, if you set your primary goal as exercising four times a week, your secondary goal would be the improved scores on your assessment. This gives you greater control. You can guarantee that you will exercise four times a week, and if you do so, you will almost certainly see the improvements you are striving for. But you have less control over the amount of improvement.

Step 3: Decide What You Need to Do   This step links your goal setting with your program development, discussed in the preceding chapters. You should think through what you need to do to accomplish your goal. Make your goals specific. For example, to meet the agency's fitness standard, you will have to exercise at least three times a week. Following your doctor's orders may require changes in diet, smoking habits, or perhaps a combination of several things. When setting your goals, also consider what resources you have to work with. For example, decide what will be the best time for exercise, what equipment you will need, and where you can find it.

Step 4: Check Your Progress   Obviously, to determine if you are making progress, you must periodically retest yourself. You want to get a feel for the effectiveness of your program and recognize if you need to change it. Set up a regular schedule for reevaluating yourself. For example, retesting every four weeks allows enough time for improvement between tests. But don't let too much time go by between tests. If you do not see improvement after four weeks, especially early on, your program is probably lacking in some way. Most likely it is the intensity with which you are exercising.

If you fail to meet your goals at the end of the evaluation period, consider the possible reasons. Did you exercise frequently enough, with the correct intensity, and for the prescribed amount of time? If you answer yes to these questions, you may have set your goals too high. Don't be discouraged.

As you learn more about your capabilities, you'll find that you can be more realistic in your goal setting. If you find after your first assessment that your initial goals were too high, adjusting them down to a more realistic level is not only acceptable but smart.

PROFILING YOUR FITNESS

You know your scores on each of the test items. But a test score (called a raw score) by itself does not have any meaning until it is compared to a norm or standard.

- A norm indicates how you scored compared to a reference group. The reference group may be the general population or a group of similar age, gender, or occupation. For example, you may be interested in how your performance compares to other law enforcement officers. The FitForce norms shown in table 3.1 represent a random sample of more than 4,000 officers from throughout the United States.

- A standard is a point score that has been identified as a performance criterion. For example, your agency may have conducted a validation study to identify minimum levels of performance. That becomes the agency standard.

To get a good picture of how your scores compare with the norms, you can create a fitness profile, a chart that will show at a glance what areas you need to improve. A Score Conversion Sheet and a Fitness Profile Sheet (page 172) are provided for you to convert your raw scores to percentiles and create your fitness profile. Take the following steps to create your fitness profile:

1. Write your raw scores for each event in the appropriate space on the Score Conversion Sheet.
2. Compare your raw scores to the FitForce norms in table 3.1 (page 39).
3. Write the closest percentile for each event in the appropriate space.
4. On the Fitness Profile Sheet, place an X where your raw score falls for each event.

SETTING GOALS USING CHAMPS

Through the years we have learned how to make goal setting more effective. These concepts are relatively simple, and to help you remember them, we developed the acronym CHAMPS. CHAMPS represents the principles of effective goal setting in that goals should be challenging, homed in, attainable, measurable, performance oriented, and should be short, mid-, and long range.

Score Conversion Sheet

Fitness area	Test	Raw score	Percentile
Cardiovascular endurance	1.5-mile run	_____	_____
Flexibility	Sit-and-reach test	_____	_____
Muscular endurance	1-minute sit-up Maximum push-up	_____ _____	_____ _____
Muscular strength	1RM bench press	_____	_____
Body composition (two options)	% fat BMI	_____ _____	_____ _____
Anaerobic power	300-meter run Vertical jump Agility run	_____ _____ _____	_____ _____ _____

From *Fit for Duty, Second Edition,* by Robert Hoffman and Thomas R. Collingwood, 2005, Champaign, IL: Human Kinetics.

Fitness Profile Sheet

Fitness area	Fitness test	FITNESS CATEGORY (percentile)		
		High 70-99	Moderate 30-69	Low 1-29
Cardiovascular endurance	1.5-mile run	_____	_____	_____

Anaerobic fitness
  Anaerobic power
  Explosive strength
  Agility
	
	300-meter run
	Vertical jump
	Agility run
		
		_____
		_____
		_____
			
			_____
			_____
			_____
				
				_____
				_____
				_____

Flexibility	Sit-and-reach test	_____	_____	_____

Muscular endurance
  Abdominal
  Upper body
	
	Sit-ups
	Push-ups
		
		_____
		_____
			
			_____
			_____
				
				_____
				_____

Absolute strength Upper body	 1RM bench press raw 1RM bench press ratio	 _____ _____	 _____ _____	 _____ _____
Body composition	% fat BMI	_____ _____	_____ _____	_____ _____

From *Fit for Duty, Second Edition,* by Robert Hoffman and Thomas R. Collingwood, 2005, Champaign, IL: Human Kinetics.

Challenging. To be effective, goals must challenge the individual. Setting a goal of losing 1 pound is not challenging and will not cause someone to maintain interest in accomplishing that goal.

Homed in. We often hear officers state goals of "getting in shape" or "toning up." Although those goals may be challenging, they are not specific enough to develop a plan of action.

Attainable. A goal of winning the Olympic marathon is challenging and homed in but is only attainable for an extremely limited group of elite endurance athletes. A more attainable goal might be to someday run a marathon.

Measurable. In addition to lacking specificity, goals such as "getting in shape" aren't necessarily measurable. A goal to become more active or change body composition is measurable.

Performance oriented. Examples of performance-oriented goals are to walk five days a week, get to the weight room three times a week, and make 10 food substitutions a week. You have complete control over accomplishing performance goals. You are probably more familiar with "outcome" goals. Examples of outcome goals would be to lose 10 pounds, improve your bench press to 225 pounds, or improve your time on the 1.5-mile run by 30 seconds. Outcome goals may be appropriate for more experienced exercisers, but beginners might be discouraged by them. For example, an officer sets a goal of losing 8 pounds in 30 days—challenging, homed in, attainable, and measurable. But in spite of increasing activity levels and consuming fewer calories, the officer loses only 6 pounds. His mind-set may be, "I did everything I was supposed to, and I failed." Officers having this experience are more apt to drop out of the program. On the other hand, if the officer's goals were to walk five days a week, lift three times a week, and make 50 food substitutions, he has complete control over whether or not he meets those goals. If he attains those goals, three things are likely to happen. One, he will lose some weight. Two, he will start developing some habits. And three, he will feel a sense of accomplishment for having successfully attained his goals.

Short, mid-, and long range. An officer who is currently running 10 miles a week sets a goal of running a marathon. It is highly unlikely for this officer to go from a long run of 2 miles to being able to complete a marathon without some intermediate goals. She might decide to plan backward from the date of the race: Be able to run 20 miles four weeks before the race; do a half marathon (13.1 miles) four months prior to the race; run 10 miles six months prior; and double the length of her long run to 4 miles, then add 1 mile a month until reaching 10 miles.

To get your creative juices flowing, the following shows how to use the CHAMPS approach for three fitness levels—low, moderate, and high.

A sedentary officer with a low level of fitness (below the 30th percentile)

Short range: Review your fitness status.

1. Record daily food intake for one week.
2. Record daily activity levels for one week. Use a pedometer to establish a baseline of daily walking.

3. Assess other lifestyle behaviors: tobacco use, substance abuse patterns, stress and weight management.

4. Calculate BMI or have body composition estimated, if possible.

Midrange: Develop and implement a plan.

1. Add 30 minutes of activity at least five of every seven days. Sample activities include walking, taking the stairs instead of the elevator, playing ball with the kids, lawn work, and gardening.

2. Make 50 food substitutions every 30 days. Sample substitutions include fish for red meat; fruits for candy, cookies, or cake; turkey for ham; water for soda; low-fat yogurt or sherbet for ice cream; and pretzels for chips.

3. Identify sources of help for other lifestyle changes (for example, smoking cessation classes, substance abuse counseling, stress management training, and weight management classes).

Long range: Turn new behaviors into habits.

1. Transition from increased activity to formal exercise. Establish a new baseline using the assessment tools in chapter 3.

2. Make food choices without thinking about it.

3. Implement other lifestyle changes as needed.

A fairly active officer with average or moderate fitness (30th to 69th percentile)

Short range: Review current fitness level and lifestyle habits. Maintain current activity level.

Midrange: Develop and implement a new plan.

1. Consider increasing frequency of exercise.

2. Run, bike, swim, or walk longer or harder, or both.

3. Increase resistance or add sets to your resistance training.

4. Add a new activity to your plan.

5. Make 15 new food substitutions per month.

Long range: Participate in a fitness competition.

1. Participate in a foot, bike, or swim race.

2. Sign up for a bench press contest.

3. Play in a three-on-three basketball tournament.

4. Play in a tennis tournament.

A regularly active officer with a high level of fitness (70th to 99th percentile)

Short range: Review current fitness status, maintaining current level of activity.

Midrange: Increase intensity of exercise or add a new activity. If applicable, make additional food substitutions.

Long range: Increase level of competition.

1. Increase race distance (performance goal).
2. Add additional activity; for example, if you are a runner, try a biathlon.
3. Improve race performance (outcome goal).

CREATING SAMPLE GOALS FOR VARIOUS FITNESS LEVELS

Some of you may be interested in establishing goals that go beyond those connected to your agency's standards. For one thing, your agency is not likely to include behavioral goals such as smoking cessation in their standards, but we know that healthy behaviors are an important part of overall fitness. You can use the Personal Inventory Worksheet below to help you evaluate your lifestyle choices in light of your fitness goals. The following list will give you more ideas for setting personal fitness goals. Use the FitForce fitness norms to help you determine how fit you are compared to other officers.

Personal Inventory Worksheet

Answer yes or no to each of the following questions.

	Yes	No
Do I need more exercise?	____	____
Would I like to look better?	____	____
Should I eat better?	____	____
Do I smoke?	____	____
Do I have more than two drinks per day?	____	____
Do I often experience stress?	____	____
Should I get more sleep?	____	____
Do I have other unhealthy behaviors?	____	____

From *Fit for Duty, Second Edition,* by Robert Hoffman and Thomas R. Collingwood, 2005, Champaign, IL: Human Kinetics.

For officers scoring at the 70th percentile and higher

Run a 10-kilometer road race.

Complete a half marathon.

Bench press 1.5 times your body weight.

Participate in a triathlon.

For officers scoring between the 50th and 70th percentiles

Complete a 5-kilometer road race.

Bench press 1.25 times your body weight.

Reduce your body fat by 3 percent.

Eliminate all yes responses on your personal inventory worksheet.

For officers scoring between the 30th and 50th percentiles

Establish a habit of working out at least three times a week for each component of fitness.

Run 3 miles without undue fatigue.

Bench press your body weight.

Reduce your body fat by 3 percent.

Reduce the number of yes responses on your personal inventory worksheet by one each quarter.

For officers scoring below the 30th percentile

Establish a habit of working out three times a week for each component of fitness.

Walk 3 miles without undue fatigue.

Improve your 1RM on each strength training exercise by 10 percent each quarter.

Reduce your body fat by 3 percent.

Reduce the number of yes responses on your personal inventory worksheet by one each quarter.

USING A GOAL-SETTING WORKSHEET

You should now be ready to set goals in a systematic way based on your fitness assessment scores. You will be using the Goal-Setting Worksheet on the following page.

To fill out the Goal-Setting Worksheet, follow these steps:

1. Make several copies of the worksheet because you will periodically reassess your goals.

2. From your assessment sheet, fill in the scores for each of the tests.

3. Once you have decided on a goal for each of the events, record it on the next line.

4. Decide how much time you are going to give yourself to achieve each goal and record it in the appropriate space. Recall the guidelines on how long it takes to achieve a training effect and time your goal accordingly.

5. Under "Other goals," enter your non-physical-fitness goals. Be specific (for example, lower your cholesterol, quit smoking, or lose 15 pounds).

6. Post a copy of your goals where you will see them several times every day. Make sure that a copy of your diet goals is visible in the kitchen.

Goal-Setting Worksheet

Instructions: Fill in your current raw scores from the nine-item fitness assessment in chapter 3. Determine your goal and the number of weeks needed to reach that goal. Enter those numbers in the corresponding blanks.

Fitness area	Current raw scores	Goal	Weeks needed to reach goal
1. Cardiovascular endurance	1.5-mile time: _____	_____	_____
2. Anaerobic fitness	300-meter time: _____ Vertical jump (inches): _____ Agility run time: _____	_____ _____ _____	_____ _____ _____
3. Flexibility	Sit-and-reach (inches): _____	_____	_____
4. Muscular endurance	Sit-ups: _____ Push-ups: _____	_____ _____	_____ _____
5. Absolute strength	Bench press (raw score): _____ Bench press (ratio score): _____	_____ _____	_____ _____
6. Body composition	% fat or BMI: _____ Current body weight: _____	_____ _____	_____ _____

7. Other goals
    Smoking cessation
    Stress management
    Control of substance abuse
			_____
			_____
			_____

From *Fit for Duty, Second Edition,* by Robert Hoffman and Thomas R. Collingwood, 2005, Champaign, IL: Human Kinetics.

To set a goal for each fitness area, use the following information as a guide. Use the FitForce fitness norms to help you determine how fit you are compared to other officers. Depending on your individual circumstances, you may want to set your goals higher or lower for each category.

- If the fitness test raw score is at the 70th percentile or higher, that means your scores are higher than 69 percent of the law enforcement population. Maintaining that level of fitness may be appropriate. The goal would be to attain the same performance on subsequent assessments.

- If you are at the 70th percentile or higher but still want to improve in one or more areas, multiply the raw score by 0.05 (5 percent). Subtract that number from the raw score for the 1.5-mile test, the 300-meter run, and the agility run. Add the 5-percent improvement number to the sit-and-reach, bench press, vertical jump, push-up, and sit-up scores.

- If the fitness test raw score is below the 70th percentile, an improvement goal is appropriate. Multiply the raw score by 0.10 (10 percent). For each test item, add or subtract the improvement number as in the preceding paragraph.

- For those who exercise regularly following the guidelines presented in chapters 5 through 8, it will take three to four weeks to achieve improvement in each component of fitness. Those who are untrained may see some improvements in shorter time periods.

- When setting the time to achieve your goals, allow enough time to ensure that there will be some improvement, but don't set times so far out that you lose interest.

- Allowing from 4 to 12 weeks between retests should accomplish your objective. Of course, this will depend on factors such as your work schedule, how faithful you are to your workout schedule, and injuries.

Goal setting is important in everything you do. It's virtually impossible to accomplish anything worthwhile if you do not know what it is you are trying to achieve. Use the information here and in the next chapter to give yourself a realistic road map to get you where you want to go and an idea of what roadblocks may get in your way.

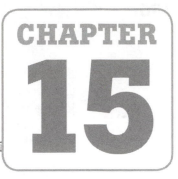
Motivating Yourself to Be Fit

As noted in preceding chapters, compliance with a fitness program is a real problem, with most adults dropping out after a few months.

Exercise

   50 percent drop out within six months to a year

   75 percent drop out within three years

Eating habits

   20 to 80 percent fail to follow a prescribed diet

   90 percent fail to reach weight-loss goals

Smoking

   60 to 90 percent go back to smoking within six months

We can conclude from these statistics that the odds are against sticking with a program.

You can do two things, however, that will help you stick with and enjoy your program. The first is to be *aware* of the slippage and dropout problem and the expectations that can affect your motivation. The second is to *act* to prevent yourself from dropping out or slipping from your program and to provide your own motivation.

"Forewarned is forearmed" is an old adage that has bearing on the potential for dropping out of exercise. You may have very high expectations or you may have a wait-and-see attitude. It can be easy to get discouraged when you don't see results as quickly as you may like, and that can get you thinking about quitting. Regardless, by being aware of several factors, you may not get so discouraged when you think about quitting.

IDENTIFYING COMMON ROADBLOCKS

Behavioral scientists have been intrigued by the problem of sticking to exercise programs and have identified some common denominators among fitness dropouts. They have categorized these characteristics as psychological, behavioral, biological, social and environmental, and programming.

Psychological factors

Low self-esteem   Apathy

High depression   Low willpower

High anxiety   Low persistence

High extroversion   Low dependability

Low expectancy of success   Low determination

Lack of self-motivation   Low organization

Behavioral factors

Inactive lifestyle   Always rushed

Smoking   Poor credit

Type A personality   Lack of ability to set goals

Biological factors

Low fitness level   Injury prone

High body fat

Social and environmental factors

Low family support   Lack of group activity support

Low peer support   Lack of organizational support

Lack of leadership   Job situation: high travel, change

Lack of cultural support

Programming factors

Inconvenient   Lack of individual prescription

Lack of leader modeling   Lack of activity variety

Lack of feedback and reinforcement   Too costly

Inflexible goals   Lack of information

Too high an activity intensity   Lack of structure

Look at the above factors and decide if you are potentially a fitness dropout. Your attitude shouldn't be that you can't overcome these obstacles. Rather, you need to be aware that sticking with the program may be tougher for you, and you must commit yourself to extra effort if you are to be successful.

Studies conducted to examine this issue have identified reasons given by those who stick with exercise and those who drop out (see Differences Between Exercisers and Dropouts below). Review those reasons and ask yourself, "Do I have a good reason for sticking with or quitting my program?"

Differences Between Exercisers and Dropouts

Why adults say they exercise	**Why adults say they drop out**
Health	No interest
Look good	Poor choice of program or facilities
Be with a group	Competing health-compromising lifestyles
Feel good	Poor perception of and attitude about exercise
Minimize aging	Poor choice of exercise mode
Have fun	Preexisting injury or illness
	No time
	No energy
	Too far out of shape
	No results
	Don't know how to get started

The three most dangerous times for potentially dropping out of your program are after the assessment, after two or three sessions, and after completing a formal program.

After the Assessment   You may feel that you are too far out of shape to make the effort worthwhile. Remember why you wanted to get started in the first place. Also remember the old Chinese proverb: "A journey of a thousand miles begins with a single step."

After Two Sessions   The first few exercise sessions may be a serious shock to your body. After perhaps years of inactivity, suddenly stressing the body can result in pain and soreness. You have to resist the temptation to do too much too soon.

After Completing a Formal Program   During a formal program, you will have support and incentives that may not exist when you are on your own. The loss of this support when the program ends can be daunting, but don't let it scare you away from continuing toward your goal of a fitter, healthier you.

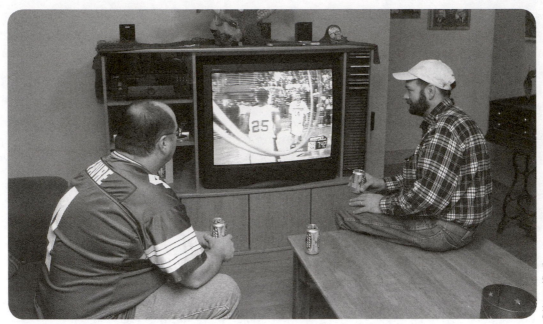

Once you've met your goals and achieved your desired fitness level, don't let yourself become inactive.

ACTING TO AVOID SLIPPING AND DROPPING OUT

Everyone has bad days, and sometimes we all need a little extra push to get out the door for exercise. Becoming aware of what you may face can help, but now you'll learn some actions you can take to avoid being a dropout statistic. If you're like most exercisers, you'll experience two levels of setback before become a dropout. Understanding what they are and how they relate to dropping out can help you avoid discouragement.

- **Slips.** All exercisers have some slips in their program. A slip is not a failure. Slips may be due to unavoidable circumstances or to laziness. In either case, although it's important to stick with your goal, recognize that a slip will not sabotage your effort. If you can make it up, do so. If not, don't think that your conditioning has been affected so seriously that further effort is useless. Just don't let your slips progress into a lapse.

- **Lapses.** When do slips become a lapse? A lapse represents a return to your former unwanted behaviors. If you have gone more than a week without exercising, for example, you may consider yourself to have suffered a lapse. Although clearly more serious than a slip, a lapse is not the end of the world either. Once again, remind yourself of why you started the program and how good you will feel when you have reached your goals. Get back on track as soon as possible to avoid becoming a fitness dropout.

- **Dropouts.** When you have dropped out, it means you have abandoned your program. You have decided that you can't do it and your goals aren't important enough for you to make the trade-offs necessary to accomplish them.

One of the major causes for dropping out of exercise is getting injured. Here are several things you can do to minimize that risk.

Warm Up and Cool Down   Following the guidelines for moving in and out of strenuous activity can go a long way toward preventing injuries.

Take a Break   If you are sick or have an acute injury, take time off and rest.

Stick With the Progression   The exercise plan as designed is set up to increase the workload or effort gradually. Trying to do too much too soon can lead to injuries.

Treatment   When you do suffer an injury, your best bet is to follow a general guideline known as RICE that, if applied immediately, will help minimize the damage. The acronym stands for the following:

Rest.

Ice the injury site.

Compress the injury site.

Elevate the injured area.

FITNESS TRAINING MYTHS

There are as many myths attributed to exercise as there are to nutrition. Knowing some of the main ones can ensure that you do not get misled into expecting too much or too little from your program.

Aerobic Exercise Is All You Need   Over the years, so much emphasis has been placed on aerobic exercise as a means of preventing health problems that some believe it is the only exercise needed. All the current research shows that maintaining a balance of aerobic, strength, and flexibility activities is necessary to get the full health benefits of exercise.

Spot Reducing Is Possible   Unfortunately, this is not true. The specific location where we gain or lose fat is genetically determined. We tend to lose weight over the entire body.

Strength Training Is Not for Women or the Elderly   Although resistance training is appropriate for everyone, how we accommodate to training is different. Neither men nor women, regardless of age, will become muscle-bound through strength training. Women do not get big gains in muscle mass because they do not have the hormone testosterone. The same holds true as we get older. We gain strength by becoming more efficient in recruiting muscle fibers.

No Pain, No Gain   You can train without having to exercise at such a high intensity that the workout causes pain. You may have temporary muscle soreness when you first start to train because the muscles are not used to activity. With reasonable goals, moderate training, and proper warm-up and cool-down, soreness can be minimized.

Exercise Increases Appetite and Weight Gain   Over time, the opposite occurs. The slight increase in food intake is more than offset by the increase in calorie utilization through exercise.

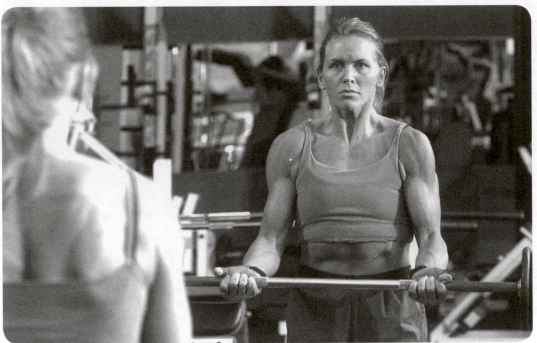

Don't be held back by myths. Everyone can benefit from physical activity.

REVIEWING YOUR PERFORMANCE

Reviewing your performance is a way to stay focused and keep your exercise a priority. It involves two major activities: (1) monitoring your exercise and (2) reassessing your fitness level, goals, and exercise and nutritional plans.

Monitoring Exercise   The simple act of keeping track of your exercise will have a positive effect on sticking with your program. A variety of exercise monitoring logs are available at fitness and sporting goods stores. For example, the Exercise Log on the following page will enable you to record your daily exercise.

Each day that you exercise, enter the type of activity, the time or duration spent on it, and whether you met the performance goals for the exercise plan (that is, the number of sit-ups or the time and distance of runs). "Practice makes perfect" is an old cliché, but one that has a bearing on adherence to exercise. It takes a minimum of three to four weeks for habits to form. Practicing your new behaviors regularly is the only way to make them become the habits you want them to be. Using a monitoring procedure is one tool for ensuring that the "practice" gets done.

Reassessing Yourself   Whether we want to admit it or not, we all have a sense of pride. Assessing our fitness level may or may not make us feel proud; however, the act of self-assessment is a necessary step for developing self-awareness, self-confidence, and self-pride. It says we are worth making the effort to look at ourselves.

The general guideline is to reassess fitness levels by retaking the fitness tests about every 12 weeks. Reviewing your goals to see if they are realistic is also important. Make modifications as necessary. If you did not reach a particular

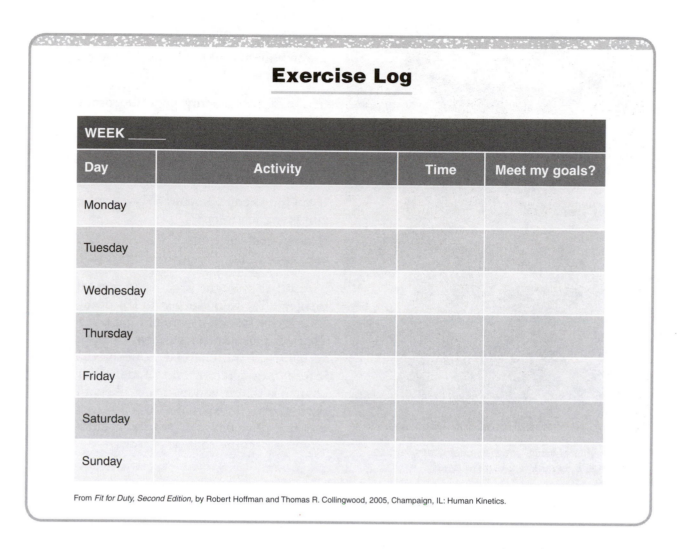

Exercise Log

WEEK _____			
Day	**Activity**	**Time**	**Meet my goals?**
Monday			
Tuesday			
Wednesday			
Thursday			
Friday			
Saturday			
Sunday			

From *Fit for Duty, Second Edition*, by Robert Hoffman and Thomas R. Collingwood, 2005, Champaign, IL: Human Kinetics.

goal, do not think of it as a failure; it only means you need to break down that goal into smaller increments. Finally, you need to review your exercise plans. The first factor to look at is the type of activity. Was it an activity you enjoyed doing? Another factor to review is the progression plan for the exercise. Were you able to follow it and meet your exercise performance goals? Reviewing your exercise log can aid in that determination. Finally, make whatever modifications you think make sense to meet your revised goals.

REWARDING YOURSELF

Another word for rewarding yourself is motivation. You can do several things to provide your own motivation, all of which are under your control.

Thought Management How you think about your exercise can influence the progress you make. There is power in positive thinking, and thinking positively can help in reaching goals. The psychological concept called the "self-fulfilling prophecy" actually works. If you think you will succeed at something, you will. Likewise, having doubts about your ability to achieve your goals decreases your chances of meeting them. Whenever negative thoughts creep in, try to reverse

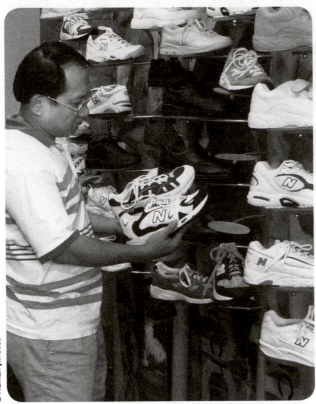

© Human Kinetics

Stick with your physical activity, meet your goals, and give yourself a reward. You worked hard!

the thinking process and say the positive statements out loud. Here are some examples:

"If I can achieve my goal" becomes "When I achieve my goal."

"I can't" becomes "I will."

"I want to quit" becomes "I can do this if I take my time."

"I am too tired" becomes "My exercise will give me energy."

"I don't have the time" becomes "I'll use some of my TV time to exercise."

Another thought process is mental imagery. Try to picture yourself doing an activity before it actually happens. That process can help prepare you to actually do the exercise. One of the interesting phenomena of behavior change is that if you try to act like a fit person, over time you perceive yourself as being physically active, and eventually you become that fit person.

Use Cues Several tips can serve as cues to keep you on course with your program:

Write the time for your exercise session on your calendar.

Put a reminder note on the refrigerator.

Have a friend or relative give you a call as a reminder.

Leave your exercise bag near the door.

Carry your exercise bag and shoes in the car.

Build in Social Support For many, the social aspect of exercising with a group is appealing. Try to associate more with individuals or groups who are exercisers. Their encouragement can be valuable support when you don't feel like exercising. Likewise, they can facilitate your making a better effort while exercising. Family and friends are another support system that can be reinforcing to your efforts. They care about you and are interested in your success, so they may be more likely to encourage your continued participation than would a group of strangers.

Build in Rewards A cardinal principle of behavior change is that having consequences for your actions is an effective way to ensure that you will stick with a new behavior. Rewards are better motivators than are punishments. You can use simple rewards to help you stay with your program. Identify both positive consequences (what you like to do, whom you like to be with, where you like to go, what you like as a special treat) and negative consequences (denying yourself the positive consequences), then build a reward system around them.

Be watchful of making the reward self-defeating, however. For example, don't reward yourself for losing 5 pounds by eating a high-calorie dessert such as a banana split or cheesecake.

Make a Contract to Exercise   Behavior contracting is a tool that combines all the motivational tips. Rewards, use of social support, and use of reminders are all incorporated into the contract. It operationalizes the commitment to exercise and serves to reinforce your efforts. A sample fitness contract is shown on page 188, along with a blank fitness contract that you can use. There are five steps to setting up a contract:

Step 1: Select a helper to help keep you honest in living up to the contract.

Step 2: Define the specifics of your exercise program in terms of what exercise routines you will do, when you will do them (days and times), and where you will do them.

Step 3: Define your responsibilities to include the cues or reminders you and your helper will use and the monitoring techniques you will use.

Step 4: Define the consequences for doing the exercise routines or not doing them. The consequences can be a combination of rewards and punishments.

Step 5: Sign the contract.

You can also use the contract as a self-contract like New Year's resolutions, where you monitor your own commitment to exercise.

You know that it is important for law enforcement officers to be fit. You also know the health risks associated with the lack of a total fitness program. You have the information you need to succeed at undertaking a fitness program that will improve your health and performance. You have learned how to set goals, how to adjust them, and how to improve your motivation. Put it all together and add the last critical ingredient—your commitment to improved health and performance. With that ingredient, you will be on the road to a longer, healthier life—for the rest of your career and as you enjoy the fruits of your labor during retirement.

Sample Fitness Contract

I will:

List the routines: Walk five times a week, do strength routine three times a week

Days and times: Walk after dinner M, T, Th, S, S, do strength routine after my shift M, W, F

Place: Walk in neighborhood, train at Bally's Gym

I will enlist the help of: My partner Joe

My responsibilities:
List reminders: Keep gym bag in car

List techniques: Keep daily log of activities

My helper's responsibilities:
List reminders: Call me before each exercise session

List techniques: Provide encouragement at every opportunity, harass me if I miss a workout

My reward for following the program:
New pair of running shoes if I do the walking for eight weeks, tickets to a ball game if I go to the gym for eight weeks

My consequence for not following the program:
Buy my partner dinner if I do not follow the program

Date: 12/4/04
Participant: John Smith
Helper: Joe Jones

Fitness Contract

I will:
List the routines: _____

Days and times: _____

Place: _____

I will enlist the help of: _____

My responsibilities:
List reminders: _____

List techniques: _____

My helpers' responsibilities:
List reminders: _____

List techniques: _____

My reward for following the program:
_____
_____

My consequence for not following the program:
_____
_____

Date: _____

Participant: _____

Helper: _____

From *Fit for Duty, Second Edition*, by Robert Hoffman and Thomas R. Collingwood, 2005, Champaign, IL: Human Kinetics.

APPENDIX

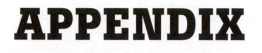

Professional Support Organizations

American Cancer Society
777 Third Ave.
New York, NY 10017
800-227-2345
www.cancer.org

American College of Sports Medicine
P.O. Box 1440
Indianapolis, IN 46206-1440
317-637-9200
www.acsm.org

American Heart Association
7272 Greenville Ave.
Dallas, TX 75231
214-373-6300
www.americanheart.org

American Hospital Association
One North Franklin
Chicago, IL 60606-3421
312-422-3000
www.hospitalconnect.com

American Lung Association
1740 Broadway
New York, NY 10019
212-315-8700
www.lungusa.org

American Red Cross
2025 E St. NW
Washington, D.C.
202-303-4498
www.redcross.com

Canadian Cancer Society
10 Alcorn Ave., Ste. 200
Toronto, ON M4V 3B1
416-961-7223
www.cancer.ca

Canadian Heart and Stroke Foundation
160 George St., Ste. 200
Ottawa, ON K1N 9M2
613-241-4361
www.heartandstroke.ca

Canadian Lung Association
1900 City Park Dr., Ste. 508
Gloucester, ON K1J 1A3
613-747-6776
www.lung.ca

Centers for Disease Control and Prevention
  (CDC)
Physical Activity and Health Branch
National Center for Chronic Disease Preven-
  tion and Health Promotion
Division of Nutrition and Physical Activity
4770 Buford Hwy. NE, MS K-46
Atlanta, GA 30341-3717
770-488-5481
www.cdc.gov

The Cooper Institute
12330 Preston Rd.
Dallas, TX 75230
972-341-3200
www.cooperinst.org

Diabetes Exercise and Sports Association
P.O. Box 1935
Litchfield Park, AZ 85340
623-535-4593
www.diabetes-exercise.org

FitForce
P.O. Box 8661
Salem, MA 01971
978-745-3629
jfitforce@aol.com

Fitness Interventions Technologies
2505 Canyon Creek
Richardson, TX 75080
972-231-8866
fittc@aol.com

Health Canada
A.L. 0900C2
Ottawa, Canada K1A 0K9
www.hc-sc.gc.ca

National Heart, Lung, and Blood Institute
National Institutes of Health
P.O. Box 30105
Bethesda, MD 20824-0105
301-592-8573
nhlbi.nih.gov

National Strength and Conditioning Association
1885 Bob Johnson Dr.
Colorado Springs, CO 80906
719-632-6722
www.nsca-fit-lift.org

Office on Smoking and Health
158 Park Bldg.
5600 Fishers Lane
Rockville, MD 20857
404-488-5705

Presidents Council on Physical Fitness and Sports
200 Independence Ave. SW
Room 738-H
Washington, D.C. 20201-0004
202-269-9000
www.fitness.gov

Thomas and Means: Law Enforcement Legal Training
P.O. Box 2039
Huntersville, NC 28070
704-895-5694
www.thomasandmeans.com

REFERENCES

American College of Sports Medicine. 2000. *Guidelines for exercise testing and prescription,* 6th ed. Philadelphia: Williams & Wilkins.

The Cooper Institute. 1990. *Health and fitness norms.* Dallas, TX: Author.

Gallup Organization. 2001. Princeton, NJ.

International Association of Chiefs of Police. 1977. *Physical fitness programs for police.* Washington, D.C.: Government Printing Office.

Landy, F. 1992. *Alternatives to chronological age in determining standards suitability for public safety jobs.* University Park, PA: Center for Applied Behavioral Sciences, Pennsylvania State University.

Law and Order. May 1994, p. 70.

Paffenbarger, R., Hyde, R., Wing, A., and Hsieh, C. 1986. Physical activity, all-cause mortality, and longevity of college alumni. *New England Journal of Medicine* 314(10): 605-613 and 315(11): 399-401.

Room, R., Barbor, T., and Rehm, J. 2005. Alcohol and public health. *Lancet* 365: 519-530.

Selye, H. 1956. *The stress of life.* New York: McGraw-Hill.

Silagy, C., Lancaster, T., Stead, L., Mant, D., and Fowler, G. 2001. Nicotine replacement therapy for smoking cessation (Cochrane Review). In *The Cochrane Library*, Issue 4. Oxford: Update Software.

USDHHS. 2000. *Healthy people 2010.* U.S. Department of Health and Human Services. Washington, D.C.: Government Printing Office.

USDHHS. 1996. *Physical activity and health: A report of the Surgeon General.* Washington, D.C.: Government Printing Office.

Wollack & Associates. 1992. *Multijurisdictional law enforcement physical skills survey.* Sacramento, CA: Author.

INDEX

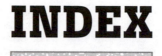

Note: The italicized *f* and *t* following page numbers refer to figures and tables, respectively.

ABOUT THE AUTHORS

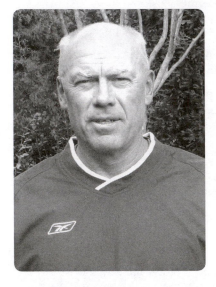

Robert Hoffman retired from the U.S. Army as a lieutenant colonel in 1991. The former director of FitForce has been training public safety officers, advising agencies about fitness issues, and helping those agencies develop fitness programs for the past 12 years. During his 22 years in the military, Hoffman completed assignments around the world. He commanded a Brigade Headquarters Company in Germany, a Ranger Company in Vietnam, and a Special Forces SCUBA Detachment at Fort Bragg, North Carolina. He also commanded the 4th Ranger Training Battalion at Fort Benning, Georgia, where in addition to working with Rangers, Hoffman trained U.S. Drug Enforcement Agents who were being deployed in South America.

Hoffman spent three years as the director of training for the Army's Soldier Physical Fitness School and helped to develop the Army's Total Fitness program. He also spent four years as a professor in the department of physical education at West Point. While there, he was an assistant cross country and track coach and a junior varsity basketball coach.

Hoffman is certified as a fitness instructor by the American College of Sports Medicine (ACSM) and as a master fitness trainer by the U.S. Army. He holds a master's degree in physical education from Indiana University and is a member of the American Society of Law Enforcement Trainers. Hoffman is also the author of *Running Together: The Family Book of Jogging*, and he helped write the army's *Physical Fitness Training* field manual. Hoffman continues to develop public safety fitness programs that are practical, effective, and legally defensible. Hoffman resides in Huntersville, North Carolina, with his wife, Barbara.